The Heart Book

About the Author

Professor Robert Kelly, MD, MBA, FRCPI, FACC, FESC, FFSEM, is a consultant cardiology and lifestyle medicine physician, associate professor of Clinical Medicine at UCD Beacon Hospital, Dublin, Ireland, honorary senior lecturer in Lifestyle Medicine, and a faculty member of the Departments of Positive Psychology and of Sports and Exercise Medicine, RCSI, University of Health Sciences Dublin, Ireland.

He is also a thought leader, author and public speaker, and certified Tiny Habits coach and behaviour designer, helping individuals, patients, health care professionals and corporates to design and adopt behaviours that transform physical, heart and emotional health and wellbeing.

The Heart Book

Making Positive Changes for a Healthy and Happier Life

Professor Robert Kelly

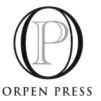

ORPEN PRESS

Published by
Orpen Press
Upper Floor, Unit B3
Hume Centre, Hume Avenue
Park West Industrial Estate
Dublin 12

email: info@orpenpress.com
www.orpenpress.com

Paperback ISBN 978-1-78605-221-6
ePub ISBN 978-1-78605-222-3

This book is designed to provide information and support to our readers. It is not intended as a substitute for professional advice from health professionals. The reader should always consult a relevant professional when required. The content of this book is the sole expression and opinion of the author. No warranties or guarantees are expressed or implied by the publisher's choice to include any of the content in this volume. Neither the publisher nor the author shall be liable for any physical, psychological, emotional, financial or commercial damages, including, but not limited to, special, incidental, consequential or other damages.

Typesetting by www.typesetting.ie
Printed in Dublin by SPRINTBOOKS

Acknowledgements

Thank you to:

My wife, Lorna, and children, Harry, Dan and Lara.
My parents, siblings, and friends.
Marie Murray, advisor and literary support.
Amy Vest, behaviour designer mentor.
BJ Fogg, behaviour designer and habits mentor.
Beth Frates, lifestyle medicine leader and mentor.
Bob Proctor Programs, personal development.
Jack Canfield, personal development mentor.
Beacon Hospital, Dublin, Ireland, home of my clinical practice.
Cardiology and Lifestyle Medicine, and colleagues worldwide.
Deirdre and Ruth at RK Cardiology.
My patients, to whom I am so grateful, for letting me into their lives and trusting me with their care.

Table of Contents

Acronyms

BMI	Body Mass Index
BP	Blood pressure
CPR	Cardiopulmonary resuscitation
COPD	Chronic obstructive airways diseases
CT	Cat scan X-ray
CVH	Cardiovascular health
ECG	Heart tracing
HCP	Health care professional
HSE	Health Service Executive
ICU	Intensive Care Unit
MRI	Magnetic resonance imaging
PFT	Pulmonary function tests
POT Syndrome/POTS	Postural Orthostatic Tachycardia Syndrome
TCM	Transtheoretical model of change

Preface

Life is short and fragile. I lost my healthy younger brother at the age of 21 to sudden cardiac arrhythmic death. This life-changing experience guided me to share my professional and personal journey in this book to inform and protect people insofar as possible from the tragedy of preventable loss.

As a professor of medicine, consultant cardiologist and lifestyle medicine doctor in Dublin, Ireland, I help to extend people's lives, I open blocked arteries in heart attack patients, and I try to prevent people dying prematurely. Stents and medications can save these lives, but the reasons why the heart events occur need to be identified and treated. These include underlying chronic conditions like smoking, diabetes, cholesterol, high blood pressure, family history, poor diet, sleep problems, stress, inactivity, isolation, and loneliness. These lifestyle factors cause heart disease, strokes, and premature death. Covid-19 has added itself to the risk list.

A healthy lifestyle can prevent, treat, and reverse chronic diseases. But that is much more difficult than inserting stents and taking medications, because it takes time and effort to do. People are aware of what to do, but despite this many seem to be unable to change health habits despite good intentions and the annual New Year resolutions, which are frequently abandoned in days.

In 2014, I added lifestyle medicine and mind–body medicine to my skill set, drawn by the opportunity to potentially cure patients beyond the pills and the stents. I realised that changing health behaviour needed a much better understanding of people, their habits and both their emotional and physical health. I realised that lifestyle changes were scientifically proven to improve heart health and I needed to learn coaching skills to communicate this to patients.

In 2017 I became a certified Tiny Habits coach and behaviour designer. This is a simple validated way to help people change behaviour and is ideal for improving heart health. It involves teaching small, practical steps that are easy and fun to do. These are explained in this book. I have also integrated these steps into my clinical practice and use them to transform people's health and wellbeing.

I enjoy meeting people, listening to their stories and how their health has evolved. Understanding the person and why they are having health concerns is a great starting step to transforming their health.

Over the last 30 years in practice, I have been drawn to helping people enjoy their best health and wellbeing. I desire the exact same for myself and everyone around me. Lifestyle medicine, having a regular check-up with a doctor and being healthy each day in your thoughts, behaviours, and habits are the keys to a healthy, successful, happy, and long life.

The second half of the book shows the reader how to make meaningful behaviour change, sustain habits, and overcome any limiting beliefs around their personal health.

At the end of the book are practical steps for sleeping better, stressing less, healthier eating and exercise tips, which I use with my cardiology patients.

I encourage you to take time when reading each chapter, to look at your own life and health and to apply these lessons to your own personal health and life story.

Read each chapter and pause, reflect what applies to your life, apply the learnings and repeat that over a few days before moving to the next chapter. Go through the tools of behaviour change slowly: pick just one, two or three behaviours to start with and get the process working for you.

Pick one big goal around your health – such as taking on more exercise – and work through the steps that suit you. If you slip, go back, and read the relevant chapters again to see where you might need to change. If nothing is happening for you, then you need to take another look at what you might be missing in your mindset and small steps. Are you able and motivated enough to make a change? Have you clear goals and a plan in place to succeed?

Enjoy your journey, have fun, and feel great in being the healthiest, best version of you every day. Share your journey with your family, friends, work colleagues and with me.

I hope that this book helps you to realise easy, practical steps to transform your health and wellbeing, and to prevent, treat and reverse chronic diseases.

I hope you learn and practice small healthy steps to keep you free from serious illness, to give you tools and the ability to deal with health scares and worries, but most of all to bring a feeling of amazing health that you want to share with others and encourage them to follow the same steps.

This book is dedicated to my wife and family, my parents (including my late father, who encouraged me for years to write this book), my siblings, my friends, my patients, my work colleagues, my clients, and everyone who has supported my efforts to transform heart health around the world. I dream of a future where the entire world chooses to be healthy each day.

Introduction

James, aged 36 years, was admitted under my care with a heart attack. Apart from treating a 28-year-old man in the US who had all his coronary arteries blocked from cocaine use, James is the youngest heart attack patient that I have come across in Ireland.

How does a 36-year-old man have a life-threatening heart attack? His mum had heart disease, but she smoked cigarettes and did not look after her health. James was healthy and had no other risk factors, with one exception: he was a director of human resources with responsibility for 5,000 employees in a big company, and he was incredibly stressed. He had two blocked arteries (out of three) and ended up with five stents and four new medications, but he was alive.

That same week, Paul, aged 37, presented to the hospital with chest pain while cycling his bike to work. He was stressed and cycled every day (to get exercise and de-stress). He was over-weight, he had two young children, and his wife was expecting their third child that same week.

Paul's angiogram showed a critical left main artery narrowing of 80 per cent severity – most people die from these blockages, known as 'widow-makers', because this artery supplies all the heart muscle from this location. Paul had one stent placed and gained a second chance at life. His initial recovery was complicated by his

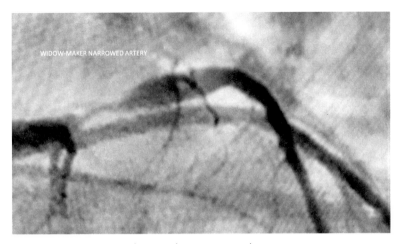

WIDOW-MAKER NARROWED ARTERY

Widow-maker narrowed artery

refusal to change his lifestyle circumstances, thinking that the stent cured him. His company introduced parental leave and this time off transformed his recovery.

I am a cardiologist, and I try to extend people's lives: by jump-starting their hearts; opening a blocked artery with a stent; slowing a racing heartbeat; detecting and treating a critical blockage on a CT scan; preventing the imminent death of the patient and thereby saving a human life, a family, a marriage, a parent, a sibling, a workmate, a friend (and the world).

However, my objective goes beyond getting a patient through the acute presentation – it includes preventing near-death from happening again. That may mean tablets, exercise, changing diet, stopping smoking, sleeping better, managing stress, and spending more time with family and friends.

Innovations in technology, medication, research, and cardiology skills have transformed heart patient survival, plus length of and quality of life. Global heart attack and stroke care systems, and connected health care, have helped to improve outcomes.

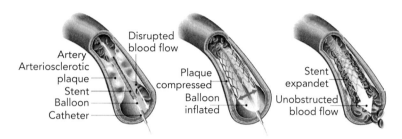

Artery disrupted blood flow

Yet in Ireland we are one of the most obese countries. There are now one billion obese people worldwide, with numbers continuing to grow in the wrong direction, meaning that a new pandemic of more Type-2 diabetes, high blood pressure, heart disease and strokes is imminent

LIVING A LONG LIFE AND AVOIDING A HEART ATTACK

The Framingham study of four family generations showed that being healthy and identifying and treating heart risk factors earlier in life leads to longevity. These actions delay the onset of heart disease by over a decade and enable people to live longer.

In some cases, patients with heart disease can live to over 100 years and many reach that milestone from a combination of these innovations and adopting a choice to live a simpler, uncomplicated, happy, healthy, and well-balanced life. Everyone will die at some point from vascular disease, cancer and/or dementia, the objective is to postpone that for as long as possible.

Healthy people can expect to live up to 80 years for men and 85 years for women. This generation are extraordinarily resilient, and commit to thrive and to enjoy life to the fullest, and they live each day this way. They want to live, and they want to enjoy it. They are rewarded for having looked after themselves throughout their eight-plus decades of life. It is worth highlighting that this generation has witnessed wars, epidemics and world recessions, and stayed strong throughout. It is fascinating to witness such resilience in so many people who were hospitalized with Covid-19 and managed to pull through.

HEALTHY AGEING

What is healthy aging? Many older people live independent, active lives, and some still drive a car at 90 years. They socialise with family and friends, and they enjoy living. Most are incredibly happy, purposeful, positive and want to keep on going. They eat small meals and drink a little alcohol. They have a daily routine and purpose. They exercise most days (looking after their physical health). They pray, go to Mass or engage in religious worship (looking after their spiritual health). They read, play bridge, do crosswords, write and a few still work. They have hobbies ranging from fishing, gardening and bridge, to horse-breeding, tennis and hillwalking, to name just a few examples. Many take a daily nap at lunchtime. All are grateful for what they have and practice that gratitude each day (looking after their emotional health).

I look after several patients in this age group. I recall one 93-year-old patient who spent the last ten years of his life using an exercise bike and treadmill on his balcony every day up to his 90th birthday. His physical health started to decline at 88 years, so he reduced the pace on the treadmill, but he continued a little exercise for a few minutes every day.

I have a 96-year-old patient who walked 500 kilometres last year around his garden by doing 2 kilometres most days. Next year he has a goal of walking 600 kilometres. I looked after a 97-year-old man with chest pain (now 103 years old) who was sent for an angiogram to investigate his heart arteries. He tried medication but his chest pain continued. I put a stent in one blocked artery, and he is alive, well, and doing his gardening and still works.

Age is no barrier for treating heart disease and these patients can go on to live even longer, happy and productive lives.

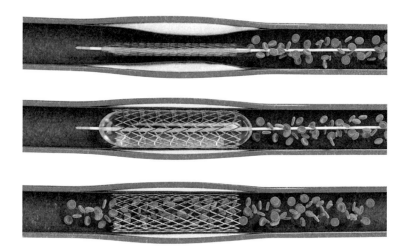

Artery stent

In these older patients, excellent quality of life is the objective of treatment. Most of these people have lived an active life for decades and this has deferred serious illness. They just want to keep going and enjoy themselves for as long as they can.

LIVING LONG AND FREE OF HEART DISEASE

Most people do not reach their 80th birthday because they fail to look after their own health and die much earlier. This happens despite all the innovations and new medications that are available in modern medicine. Those interventions alone cannot cure physical illnesses like heart disease, strokes or cancer. Having a stent or surgery extends your health span by decades *if* you also take medications, follow up, have regular blood work, *and* undo all the reasons why you have a heart problem. Failing that, you will need more stents or even have to redo surgery, or in several cases you may not survive to have these options.

Patients frequently think that stents make their heart problem disappear. Many patients belong to this category: some will not take medications as instructed, others not all medications, others will eat, smoke and stress believing that medications will keep their problems away. Cholesterol tablets do reduce the risk of disease progression but not without changing diet and removing other risk factors, like stopping smoking, managing stress and sleep, and taking exercise.

It has always fascinated me as to why we as doctors are not curing heart disease. Patients ask 'Can you not dissolve the plaque blocking arteries that causes strokes and heart attacks? Are there no pills to cure all illnesses?'

I ask:

'Are we trying to tackle the problems like heart attacks at the wrong end, namely treatment, instead of the root cause, or understanding why the artery has blocked, or why has this person developed a problem, and can we do something different? We already do so much and yet heart disease remains the number one cause of premature death – are we doing this wrong/are we looking in the wrong place?'

I have come across several ways to prevent and even regress heart disease. Anyone who wants to, can reach a healthy, flourishing big age milestone if they choose to live a simpler, purpose-filled, less stressful, healthy, happy and more balanced lifestyle. The challenge for healthy longevity is empowering patients to commit to a healthier way of living.

The NHS has a useful tool for calculating your heart age, which can be accessed on www.nhs.uk/health-assessment-tools/calculate-your-heart-age. I urge everyone to go online and complete it to get a better understanding of your heart health.

THE REALITIES OF HEART DISEASE

Heart disease is the leading cause of premature death worldwide (29 per cent) and sadly the numbers continue to rise. Heart disease is caused by genes, high blood pressure, diabetes, high cholesterol, obesity, smoking, drug misuse and alcohol. Those causes result from the way we live our lives: poor sleep, stress, poor eating behaviours, physical inactivity and loneliness/isolation from friends and family. Genes account for 10–20 per cent of risk.

Despite that, most patients with a family history of heart disease make excuses about a relative's heart problems as a lifestyle issue, so they themselves do not come forward to get their own health risk checked out. In truth, poor health is due to human behaviour in 50 per cent of cases, environment in 20 per cent, access to care in 10 per cent, and genes in 20 per cent of cases. Yet we focus on access to hospitals without addressing 70 per cent of the causes for chronic ill health, most of which are preventable.

Recent headlines in the United States report that less than 5 per cent of Americans are healthy! Three-quarters are overweight or obese, and about 50 per cent have diabetes or pre-diabetes. Adults with diabetes are two to three times as likely to die of heart disease or stroke as those without diabetes; one in three US adults will die of heart disease or stroke; 50 per cent of US adults have chronic kidney disease, and almost 10 per cent of adults have cancer. Eighty per cent of COPD cases are caused by smoking and COPD is the fourth leading cause of death. One in three people die from Alzheimer's disease.

The same risk factors increase the mortality and morbidity of Covid-19 patients twelve-fold. High blood pressure, obesity, diabetes and smoking also increase stroke and heart attack risks in Covid-19 patients.

SUDDEN CARDIAC DEATH

One person dies every 36 seconds in the United States from heart disease. There are 10,000 deaths each year in Ireland from heart disease. Fifteen to twenty per cent of all deaths worldwide are due to sudden cardiac death and heart rhythm abnormalities. If a patient is fortunate enough to have symptoms and immediately call an ambulance there is a chance to save their life. If they collapse and early resuscitation and defibrillation shock to the heart are performed, then 10 per cent of these people may survive.

In the last fifteen years standardised pathways of emergency care have been implemented worldwide to give heart attack patients the best chance to be treated quickly and survive. Ireland has seen the benefits of this strategy.

Every year there are about 6,000 heart attacks admitted to Irish hospitals. Five per cent (2.8 per cent for those who receive primary angioplasty) die in hospital (which has improved from almost 7 per cent over ten years with this rapid angioplasty treatment approach). This compares favourably with world figures of 7 per cent for death shortly after a heart attack. In some parts of the world this figure is over 60%!

Survival rates for cardiac arrest patients are less than 10 per cent in terms of successful resuscitation and transport to hospital. Subsequent survival to discharge from hospital has improved to 13.3 per cent. In patients who are delayed in getting to hospital, the mortality rates are much higher. Out of hospital death rates vary.

In China there are more than 230 million people with heart disease and 550,000 experience cardiac arrest every year. This shows that very few people will survive a big heart attack or if their heart stops suddenly. In other cases, permanent brain damage may occur after prolonged resuscitation efforts.

SUDDEN ARRHYTHMIC DEATH SYNDROME

Premature/sudden cardiac death can also happen to younger people, usually as result of a birth defect in the heart or an undetected electrical problem. The human heart grows normally up to 30 years of age, and so it can be difficult to detect abnormalities that lead to sudden death. This particular patient population is one group where prompt treatment with CPR (resuscitation) and defibrillator use can save a life, and treatment with newer technology like implantable defibrillators can extend life.

Some of these patients may have lifestyle issues such as alcohol and drug misuse (cocaine, marijuana, ecstasy, heroin) to trigger heart problems but, in general, the majority do not have identifiable causes for the sudden death and prevention is an ongoing scientific challenge.

This book focuses on the patients aged over 30 years who acquire heart disease related to their lifestyle. Over 30 years is an important reference because the Global Burden of Disease Review for 2019 reported an increasing prevalence of heart disease in this age group, particularly among young men.

I have treated multiple patients in their thirties and forties with exertional chest pain and no risk factors, but subsequently have discovered that work stress, smoking and diet were issues. These are people who have had critical life-threatening blockages in their arteries. They were treated with stenting, medications, lifestyle interventions and are doing well today. A handful have required coronary artery bypass surgery. Sadly, a growing number of patients have died prematurely. A few have been extraordinarily lucky to have their heart stop with a doctor standing beside them who has shocked their heart and resuscitated them. In most cases these people have a blocked artery at the front of the heart.

It is crucial to understand that no one is immune from getting heart disease or even having a heart attack. In fact, a Danish CT study of all-comers would suggest that 60 per cent of men and

40% of women have plaque in their coronary arteries. There is a high follow-up event risk (over 10 per cent) of heart attacks seen in those without heart plaque due to untreated risk factors. Sadly, many of these patients (especially men) will never come to see a doctor.

PREVENTING CARDIAC DEATH

The only way to avoid or delay heart disease is prevention: healthier choices need to be embedded earlier in life, ideally from birth. Society must wake up and value health. This links with social health prescriptions to engage the community in being healthy by activities such as walking groups, healthy eating clubs, financial and social supports, buddy services to look after neighbours, and health education and promotion. Initiatives in the UK involve link workers at GP surgeries connecting patients with those options which in most cases get to the root of, and thereby treat, the health problem. The Royal Mail has teamed up with the NHS in the UK to support community care services for patients.

Critical time windows define life: from the prenatal stage, to post-natal, in the family and at preschool, school, college, the workplace, early adulthood, into the work community, then the wider community, health and in the neighbourhood. This starts with early childhood and progresses to older age. It is important to meet people where they are on this timeline and to support every member of the community.

Smart initiatives in the United States have met people where they go: such as at church or in the hairdressers. These sites run blood pressure (BP) checks and treatment programmes which have been clinically validated and shown to be effective. In the United States there is funding to support this broadminded approach to caring for the health of the community. In the UK, barber shops have started to offer mental health counselling to customers.

There is enormous need to educate everyone (from birth, and both parents and children) in all aspects of health, emphasising the positives of health and encouraging play and physical activity, healthy approaches to stress and, most importantly, having fun in life, and valuing health and life over work and pressure. If people feel well, share and connect with others, their health will improve.

Community and friendship are important to help Covid-19 patients recover. During the pandemic, no visitors were allowed into hospital to help their loved ones to battle illness. Several ICUs resorted to using video links for patients to talk with their families. This positive support helps patients to be strong and to better fight their illness.

Living a life that you want, free of all serious preventable illnesses and postponing death and illness beyond 80 years of age, is your choice. While this may not seem relevant to most younger people, understanding what you want in life will help build your future focus on how to get there. Promoting fun is where the focus should be to get people doing things because the easier and more enjoyable human behaviour is, the more likely it will become habitual.

SECTION ONE

Heart Health

.

1

Everyday Heart Problems

HEART DISEASE AND STROKES

Heart disease causes 29 per cent of premature deaths worldwide. There were seventeen million deaths, 330 million years of life lost and thirty-six million years of life lived with disability worldwide in 2017. It is projected that heart disease will cause more than twenty-three million deaths globally by 2030. The number of strokes and deaths due to stroke has increased despite reduced numbers of strokes among older people. The fastest growing reason is explained by increased body weight. Today heart disease (and stroke) is responsible for a significant reduction in quality of life, life expectancy and imposes huge costs on health systems worldwide.

COVID-19

After a steady decline from 2010 to 2019, heart disease rates rose significantly worldwide with the onset of the Covid-19 pandemic in 2020. This represents five years of lost progress among all adults and ten years of lost progress among black adults and younger adults. Covid-19 disrupted many aspects of daily life, including access to preventative heart care which may have delayed detection and treatment of disease. In Ireland, almost two million cases of Covid-19 have been diagnosed, with 9,366 deaths.

Looking after Covid-19 patients has been a mixed experience of patient care, ranging from heroic survivors to healthy unfortunate sufferers who died or were left with permanent lung damage, new heart failure and/or disabling strokes. Several people fought their illnesses at home and were more afraid to go to hospital. This has been a truly traumatic experience for many. I recall a couple who attended for blood pressure management and told me the story of their Covid illness: both looking at each other at the kitchen table, barely able to breath, holding hands and praying to survive. Six months later they suffer with daily post-traumatic stress of near death as they sit down for breakfast.

There is growing evidence to suggest that people who had Covid-19 may be at increased risk of new or worsening heart disease. Behaviour factors such as smoking, inactivity and increased alcohol use all contributed to higher cardiovascular death rates. Increased rates were especially evident among black people, the Hispanic population, indigenous individuals and those in poorer communities.

Various heart abnormalities have been encountered in hospitalised Covid-19 patients. These include elevated biomarkers of muscle injury and heart failure, ECG abnormalities, clots, heart attacks and strokes. Some patients have experienced persistent cardiac symptoms leading to a diagnosis of prolonged Covid-19 illness.

Covid-19 has not gone away and there are thousands of people who have a long-term chronic illness from the physical damage caused by Covid-19, such as strokes, heart failure, heart attacks and long-term Covid-19 symptoms, or so-called Long Covid illness. This epidemic has left a huge psychological impact on society and increased the burden of future physical and mental illness.

Covid-19 has had significant effects including:

4

- Increased physical inactivity (50 per cent reduction in physical activity)
- Psychological impacts (20 per cent rise in suicide risk)
- Stress, isolation and loneliness, leading to a 30 per cent increase in the chance of premature death
- A 20–60 per cent increase in sleep issues
- More anxiety and depression
- Poor lifestyle choices have increased in terms of poor eating habits, sugar consumption, and increased alcohol consumption (30 per cent increase in Europe)
- Significant increase in mobile phone usage and time spent on internet, at the expense of getting outside and socialising

This is despite reports of higher death rates from Covid-19 among obese, inactive, unhealthy, and older people. Already unhealthy people have picked up more unhealthier habits.

Covid-19 has caused:

- Heart failure
- Lung clots
- Atrial fibrillation
- Heart attacks
- Strokes
- Generalised inflammation

It has triggered five times more cases of postural orthostatic tachycardia syndrome (POTS). The latter produces symptoms akin to the traditional chronic stress response, with changes in blood pressure and fast heart rates. The ongoing psychological injuries have made POTS more symptomatic for many (including fast heart beats and dizzy spells accompanied by exhaustion and brain fog).

Long Covid illness

Several people who had a Covid-19 illness have ongoing symptoms months after their initial infection, so-called 'Long Covid' illness. This has been debilitating for a previously healthy patient group. This has resulted in forced absenteeism, chronic illness, brain fog and significant mental health issues.

Long Covid is defined as persistence of Covid-19 symptoms beyond twelve weeks. Those symptoms include:

- Exertional fatigue
- Chronic fatigue
- Shortness of breath
- Palpitations
- Dizziness
- Brain fog
- Poor concentration
- Exhaustion
- Chest pain

These patients have a wide spectrum of illness, and they represent almost 10 per cent of Covid-19 sufferers across the world. Many are young, previously very fit women.

The cause of Long Covid is not clear but it may be a post-viral, inflammatory, persistent viral, endothelial dysfunction (a non-obstructive coronary artery disease (CAD) in which the large blood vessels on the heart's surface constrict (narrow) instead of dilating (opening)), impaired exercise metabolism, mitochondria energy depletion, autonomic dysfunction, or cardiac deconditioning abnormality.

Other post-viral illnesses or chronic fatigue syndrome and ME describe similar symptoms, specifically fatigue despite a night's sleep, chronic fatigue, and post-exertion malaise of over six months duration.

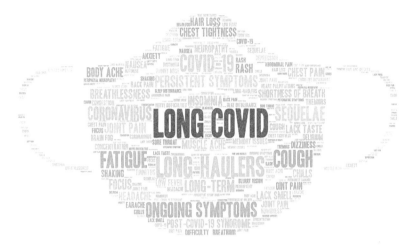

The medical assessment is symptom and story based. Physical tests may or may not be abnormal, such as myocarditis on a cardiac MRI or abnormal lung function on pulmonary testing (PFT).

Treatment is supportive of symptoms with additional medications to help with sleep, energy and brain fog as well as resolute Long Covid rehabilitation programmes. There are insights to be gained from treatments for ME and post-viral illnesses. A recent US neurology study has found that Covid-19 patients who experienced adverse life events or increased stress in their recovery were more likely to develop Long Covid illness. This identifies a potential value for behaviour approaches to support patient recovery and rehabilitation and to prevent Long Covid.

As time moves on, the after-effects of Covid-19 persist: the disease is still active worldwide with a risk of further breakouts; there is reluctance to wear masks or to get vaccinated; and the collective impact of everything is multiplying stress levels for everyone. This is added to by a recession, energy crisis, climate change, war and general catastrophizing mood. Some people have been unable to change their Covid-19 behaviours – one example is older people who are still afraid to leave their homes or go to shops for fear of getting sick. I have seen first-hand how this isolation triggers heart complaints.

RISK FACTORS THAT CAUSE HEART DISEASE

The Interheart study of over 10,000 heart attack patients found that risk factors (smoking, diet, blood pressure, cholesterol, diabetes, family history and inactivity) accounted for 80 per cent of risk.

In the Chicago Heart Project, over 30 years, the incidence of heart or stroke disease was found to be rare in patients with no risk factors. The British Heart Foundation heart risk score in patients under 50 years of age shows that if you have fewer than two heart disease risk factors, there is a 2 per cent future heart attack risk, compared with 65 per cent risk if you have more than two risk factors.

The main risk factors for heart disease are:

- High levels of LDL cholesterol, Lipoprotein (a) and ApoB lipo-protein (markers of increased cholesterol risk to heart disease)
- High blood pressure
- Cigarette smoking
- Obesity
- Diabetes
- Family history of heart disease

High blood pressure causes 9.4 million deaths and 7 per cent of global disability-adjusted life years. Smoking is responsible for 50 per cent of all the avoidable deaths in smokers, with half of these due to heart disease, stroke and vascular problems. A lifetime smoker has a 50 per cent probability of dying due to smoking and on average will lose at least ten years of life. Second-hand smoke is associated with an increase in heart disease.

The American Heart Association has defined a new construct of cardiovascular health (CVH) to promote a change in basic assumptions from a focus solely on disease treatment to one inclusive of positive health promotion and preservation across life course in populations and individuals.

That change in basic assumptions identifies eight life essentials as the principal risks to heart health:

- Physical activity
- Smoking
- Sleep health
- Body weight
- Cholesterol
- Blood glucose
- Blood pressure
- Healthy diet

They acknowledge that stress and the social determinants of health underline the foundation of all CVH. The prevalence of ideal CVH is less than 1 per cent for all age groups studied in the United States, including as young as twelve years old. The heritability of CVH is low, indicating that behavioural and environmental exposures determine CVH. These figures can be applied in a worryingly analogous manner across the world.

Diabetes

Diabetes doubles the risk for heart disease. Women with diabetes have a higher stroke risk. These patients tend to have high blood pressure and high cholesterol levels which increases the risk of heart disease and strokes to a higher level.

Obesity

Obesity or BMI over 25kg/m^2 increases all-cause mortality. Waist circumference is predictive of diabetes and heart disease. Obesity is a multi-factorial chronic disease contributed to by lifestyle behaviour, genetics, hormones, medications and social/commercial determinants of health. There are now one billion obese people worldwide.

Advancing age

Age is a major driver of risk. Being aged 40 is associated with lower risk; however, heart disease can still occur, including heart attacks. Conventional risk factors at that age sharply increase longer-term heart disease risk.

Fifty-two per cent of women over 45 years have hypertension and 40 per cent have cholesterol problems. The highest risk for major heart disease is in men over 60 and women over 75 years.

Heart disease mortality increases by 2 per cent in men over 62 years of age, usually around retirement.

In the US, those who have good CVH with five metrics (out of eight) at the ideal levels comprise:

- 55 per cent of adolescents
- 32 per cent of adults aged 20–39 years of age
- 11 per cent of adults 40–59 years of age
- 4 per cent of adults above 60 years of age

There are significant variations by race, gender and socioeconomic status, especially in younger age groups.

According to the World Health Organization, 70 per cent of global chronic diseases are due to lifestyle issues. The prevalence of an unhealthy lifestyle is high and heart disease risk factors are often poorly treated, even in patients considered to be at substantial risk.

Ireland is among one of the unhealthiest countries in the world when defined by eating habits, body mass and stress. We fare better with physical activity. Studies show that:

- 75 per cent of the world's population are chronically dehydrated
- 35 per cent sleep under seven hours per night
- 10 per cent eat a healthy recommended diet
- 25 per cent achieve the daily physical activity target
- 60 per cent are stressed
- 60 per cent are experiencing loneliness

Studies from the Mayo Clinic, USA in 2018, show that just 2.7 per cent of the US population lives a healthy lifestyle as defined by diet, regular daily exercise, not smoking and having BMI below 25.

The leading causes of death and disability worldwide are due to poor diet, lack of exercise, smoking and excess alcohol intake, stress and sleep issues.

Physical activity

- Physical inactivity increases the risk for early death, colon cancer, heart disease, breast cancer, stroke, Type-2 diabetes, hypertension and metabolic syndrome.
- Physical inactivity is a major risk factor for disease, with 50–60 per cent of the population affected (compared with 18 per cent affected by smoking, 30 per cent by bad cholesterol or 29 per cent by high blood pressure).
- Inactivity causes 11 per cent of premature mortality (5.3 million deaths worldwide, compared with 5.1 million smoking-related deaths).
- Prolonged sitting is associated with higher all-cause mortality, including heart disease, strokes and cancer.
- Remember that sitting includes working at your desk all day without taking any breaks.

Chronic stress

Chronic stress is the combined physiological and psychological impact on a person in response to adverse events or perceived events. Stress is the fight or flight response and is essential to human survival.

Burnout is a syndrome conceptualised as resulting from chronic workplace stress that has not been successfully managed. It has three dimensions:

- Feeling exhausted
- Increased mental distance from one's job
- Feelings of negativism or cynicism towards one's job and reduced professional efficacy

Stress increases risk for heart disease, stroke and cancer. It also increases the risk for lung disease, liver illness, STDs, mental health illnesses, autoimmune disorders and metabolic syndrome. It leads to absenteeism, poor work performance and premature death. In a 30-year US study of individuals without known heart disease, chronic stress was independently (of traditional heart risk factors like blood pressure, weight, cholesterol, smoking) associated with a 14 per cent increased risk of heart problems over a four-year follow-up. Stress causes hypertension, raised cholesterol, reduced immunity, memory difficulties due to poor concentration, fertility issues and mental health problems. Loneliness and isolation cause similar health problems.

Stress at work comes from:

- Workplace environment
- Poor supervision
- Management
- Workload
- Long hours
- Personal life crises

- Trauma
- Exhaustion
- Health issues
- Communication difficulties
- Relationships
- Low job autonomy
- Poor leadership
- Dysfunctional teams
- Poor team dynamics
- Lack of job satisfaction

These stresses lead to poor individual wellbeing, inferior quality interpersonal relationships and, in health care, that affects the safety and quality of patient care.

Burnout drives binge drinking, insomnia and fatigue, which trigger heart health risks and premature death.

The problems do not end here as most people seem unable to recuperate and recover after stressful days only to generate an even higher stress burden on subsequent days.

Unhealthy eating

Ireland is one of the most obese populations across Europe. Obesity is a condition that contributes to multiple diseases and comorbidities.

- It affects surgical outcomes.
- It leads to high rates of cancer, heart disease, strokes, and falls – the four most common causes of death above 50 years of age in men and women.

High sugar consumption increases cardiovascular death risk by almost 40 per cent. Alcohol and fizzy drinks contain high sugar content.

In the United States, more Americans are sick than are healthy:

- 50 per cent have diabetes or pre-diabetes
- 75 per cent are overweight or obese
- Only 10 per cent are metabolically healthy
- 25 per cent of teenagers are overweight or obese
- 20 per cent have pre-diabetes and 12 per cent have severe fatty liver disease

In 2017, 11 million deaths were attributable to dietary risk factors. High salt intake, low whole grain intake, and low fruit intake are the leading dietary risk factors for death around the world.

High cholesterol, specifically non-HDL cholesterol, is associated with cardiovascular risk. The target is total cholesterol less than five mmol/L (four if intermediate risk/plaque) and then LDL cholesterol below three mmol/L and lower is better.

Poor quality sleep

- Sleeping for less than five hours or more than nine hours increases the risk of heart attacks by 25–34 per cent.
- Insufficient sleep leads to more car accidents (22 per cent).
- Sleep is an essential element of human biology and life. It affects every physiological system.
- Poor sleep drives all-cause mortality due to cardiometabolic health.
- It affects blood pressure, glucose, and inflammation. Slight changes in sleep may lower the risk for heart disease.
- In truth, issues with sleep are multidimensional and relate to sleep duration, time, regularity, efficiency, satisfaction and impact on daytime alertness. Each of these impacts heart health.

- Poor sleep affects psychological health and social determinants of health. In fact, poor sleep may mediate those effects.
- Poor sleep doubles the risk of suicide. Uninterrupted sleep of six to eight hours is recommended for all adults over 18 years age.
- Disrupted sleep pattern increases the risk for weight gain among women, in fact good sleeping habits help you to lose weight.
- Poor sleep may be due to other medical conditions such as sleep apnoea (snoring, stopping breathing during sleep).
- Sleep apnoea is a major cause of high blood pressure and heart problems.

Addictions

- Smoking doubles your risk of having a heart attack or a stroke, and it causes 25 per cent of heart-related deaths.
- Drinking more than the recommended weekly alcohol intake (eleven units for women, fourteen for men) increases risk of stroke, diabetes, blood pressure, heart failure, obesity and heart attacks. There is a 23 per cent increased risk of a heart event for every unit drank above fourteen units among 40- to 70-year-old people at a seven-year follow-up. Functional brain MRI images show that similar increases in alcohol intake led to premature brain ageing.
- Drugs such as cannabis and cocaine are toxic for your heart.
- Cocaine increases risk of sudden death, cardiac arrhythmias, heart attacks and heart failure. Even one dose of cocaine can cause these events.
- Cannabis increases the risk of atrial fibrillation which causes strokes, heart failure, and sudden death.

2

Doctor, How Healthy Is My Heart?

The physical side of heart health is assessed and measured from:

- Patient story: past, present, future goals
- Physical examination – appearance, colour, blood pressure, heart rate, temperature, breathing, listening to chest and heart
- ECG/electrocardiogram heart tracing
- Lung function tests
- Echocardiogram – heart function, valves ultrasound scan
- Exercise stress test/treadmill
- Stress echocardiogram
- CT coronary angiogram (non-invasive imaging of arteries with CT scan)
- Invasive coronary angiogram/FFR/stent/CABG surgery
- Cardiac MRI (heart imaging in magnetic tunnel)
- Blood work – depends on each patient story and test findings
- Basic blood work – FBC, U&E, TFTs, LFTs, cholesterol, Lpa, homocysteine, Ca, Mg, PO4, BNP, vitamin levels, selenium, PSA, viral titres
- Advanced – genetic risk assessment, microbiome testing

The test results are reviewed along with the history and examination findings to predict risk for heart disease, stroke, premature death and then to find a precise way to treat and manage patients, which invariably require combined interventions of behaviours, medications, and stents/surgery.

The objective of care is a healthy patient in a healthy functioning body, free of acute risks and working for long-term freedom from disease/ill health. An opportunity to reverse damage and live a longer, healthier life is desired.

Imaging and physiology testing will inform the need for medication/stents/surgery. Precise information can help focus on lifestyle areas of greatest priority for a patient to start with or to prevent future illness, like premature ageing, stroke risk, Alzheimer's risk as examples.

Coaching is needed to optimise patients' results, to design programmes and to monitor patients' progress, help them deal with problems and address stress and other health domains. The Australian COACH program shows statistically significant improvement in heart health with this approach in patients at risk for heart attacks.

THE SCIENCE OF HUMAN DISEASE

The human body is made up of cells, organs, blood vessels, electrical systems, software and a brain computer. These work together. However, changes to one component can affect every part, for example blocking a blood vessel can shut down the computer to cause a stroke; messing with the electrical system, such as during stress, can pressurise the blood vessels and fire up the cells to release chemicals, hormones and cytokines that leak into the system and cause chaos in the form of heart attacks or strokes, or stay there and gradually eat away at the system to cause cancer. Putting dirty petrol in the system in the form of food, alcohol, drugs will break it. Not letting system rest/recharge after overworking will also break the system.

The computer is your brain and the electrical system includes nerves, neurohormones and chemicals in the brain that connect to the rest of the body via the autonomic nervous system (the wires). The latter is responsible for fight or flight or controlling how the body responds to pressure or surviving. The autonomic nervous system affects all organ functions, including heart rate and blood pressure, breathing, waterworks, metabolism, sleep and appetite.

The blood vessels carry chemicals, hormones and waste around the body to different organs. Organs have multiple functions including making repairs to the body, regenerating blood cells, fighting infection and clearing waste. These make up all body functions. Interestingly, Covid-19 seems to target the autonomic nervous system causing heart palpitations, blood pressure issues and it is thought to contribute to brain fog. Treating autonomic dysfunction can improve these symptoms and help patients with Long Covid to recover.

At a cellular level different processes link every illness. This is not fully understood. However, inflammation is the centerpiece, and it causes all diseases, albeit in separate ways. Cancer is different from heart disease but similar lifestyle behaviours like smoking can cause both conditions. It varies from person to person.

Inflammation is usually protective, like the fight or flight response, but if it is prolonged or abused (diet, stress, infection, inactivity, exhaustion) it will persist and lead to disease. Chemicals, hormones and neurotransmitters are released from different organs and carried in blood vessels. They cause inflammation as well. Increased cortisol and lower serotonin affect mood.

The science behind Covid-19 is interesting in this context: clotting, inflammation and autonomic dysfunction are key processes that affect the human body after Covid-19 and may persist in Long Covid. These affect different organs in different people, e.g. balance/hearing issues, GI issues or more commonly exhaustion, heart and lung problems.

Inflammation of heart muscle (myocarditis) is one feature. Inflammation itself triggers other consequences such as bleeding, strokes, heart attacks, autonomic dysfunction and POT Syndrome. Interestingly, many other viral illnesses cause similar effects.

Cardiovascular health (CVH) is influenced by pathways involved in inflammation, endothelial dysfunction, atherosclerosis, cardiac stress and remodelling, hemostatic factors, and epigenetics. CVH is uniquely positioned as a health outcome itself related to upstream genetic, social, behavioural and environmental factors and as a determinant of major downstream health outcomes.

Many human body systems can repair themselves and reverse early disease states. The brain can be reprogrammed and it adapts (neuroplasticity). Stroke patients report recovering from paralysis by relearning how to exercise (like learning to walk as a child).

The heart and brain are closely aligned through the autonomic nervous system and hormonal pathways.

The heart can heal by changing lifestyle, less stress, healthy foods, exercise and sleep, all of which reduce inflammation, regulate the autonomic nervous system and stabilize chemical secretions.

Meditation, conscious breathing, mindfulness, yoga and tai chi similarly regulate the autonomic nervous system and relax and calm the mind and the rest of the body.

OPTIMAL HEART HEALTH

The benefits of good heart health (CVH) show that living the highest possible levels of CVH leads to the best outcomes. The preferred approach is to change one risk at a time. The earlier in life that CVH is optimised, the better the outcomes. Optimal CVH means 50 per cent lower risk of cardiovascular disease events. Optimal CVH is associated with better long-term health outcomes at every age and improving CVH with time is associated with a reduction in heart disease of two million deaths per year.

Better CVH also means less cancer, dementia, chronic kidney disease, COPD, Alzheimer's disease, and quality of life. It also reduces mortality and morbidity seen with Covid-19 illness.

- Pursuing and sustaining a healthier lifestyle from teenager years is the best strategy for achieving higher CVH into middle age.
- The ability to choose a healthy lifestyle across your life's course is strongly influenced by psychological health factors and social plus structural determinants of health and disease.
- Younger people will often choose to exercise, but eating, sleeping, alcohol, drug misuse and stress are not dealt with.
- Recent studies show that lifestyle in the early years predict premature heart disease in mid-life.

A healthy body is a balance between good lifestyle choices regarding eating, drinking, activity, sleep and stress versus not-so-good behaviours. If the see-saw tips into bad choices, then there is a consequence. If those choices are weighed down by existing bad behaviours, then heart disease risks are higher.

Everyone is different and we don't know why. Some people have heart attacks and others do not. The reason why 80 per cent of heart attacks happen are well known and are largely prevent-able by whole health measures. Understanding the science of the human body helps us to see how various parts are linked to having a heart attack, stroke or death by inflammation pathways. This is driven by lifestyle, genes, behaviour and environment.

How we respond to these factors determines health risk. If stressed, we can breathe and switch the brain to silent, calm the mind, take breaks to rest the autonomic nervous system and reduce the cortisol levels driving the inflammation. Over time this heals the body and prevents heart disease and chronic illness, if accompanied by changing other lifestyle pillars.

In the longer term, adopting a healthier lifestyle can undo disease and delay relapse. Exercise, healthy eating and stopping smoking reduce and regress atherosclerosis, improve cancer outcomes and reduce recurrence. There may be a need for medications to help. Then it is a matter of being healthy and happy in mind and body every day.

HEALTH MODELS

Health is defined by the World Health Organization (WHO) as personal, professional, emotional, spiritual, mental, financial and physical health and not merely the absence of disease. These key areas in life combine to affect your health. This might include stress from financial worries leading to relationship issues causing heart problems and/or giving rise to heavy smoking and overeating, also causing heart problems.

The American Heart Association's cardiovascular health (CVH) model posits that social-ecological factors also affect the ability to optimise heart health. These include culture, environment, community resources, organisation networks, and individual genetic and behaviour factors. These collaborate with an individual's psychological health and provide context for what is possible to improve heart health. There is an interplay between the heart, the mind and the body connections. It is important to see the importance of these factors and their effect on health activities.

Lifestyle choices are critically important. A balanced approach better serves personal health instead of choosing extreme unintentionally risky behaviours – taking up mountain-biking in middle age after years of stress, weight gain and overeating without having your health checked out first is a recipe for health problems like heart attacks. I have seen these people having heart rhythm problems, heart attacks, sometimes a stroke from extreme exercise in the gym and near sudden death after long-distance running and cycling events.

People are working even longer hours and giving up any previously positive health behaviours such as exercise, healthy eating and sleeping. They are stressed, drinking more, smoking and the long hours are now cyclical, like a treadmill. This increases the risk of premature heart attack.

3

Can I Improve My Heart Health?

A cure is an end to a medical condition or suffering: the state of being healed. It can be achieved with medication, a procedure, a change in lifestyle or a philosophical mindset. It may mean a combination of all of these as with heart disease.

The concept of cure has evolved in cancer medicine to include immunotherapy for malignant melanoma that can stop disease progression without surgically removing the tumour. Recent studies show that resistance-based exercises halt prostate cancer progression. Whole-food, plant-based and Mediterranean diets also lower cancer risk.

Heart disease progression can be reduced with cholesterol medications, but patients also need to change their lifestyle behaviours to stop heart disease from progressing. The Ornish Lifestyle Programme of whole food plant-based eating, exercise and stress management reduces the progression of and, in some cases, reverses heart disease.

Evidence based lifestyle therapeutic approaches to prevent, treat and potentially reverse lifestyle-related chronic diseases; it is doctor delivered.
It is application of medical, behavioral, motivational, environmental principles in a clinical setting. Teaches self care management.
<u>**Pillars**</u>
Address (stop smokig / alcohol in moderation)
Nutrition
Physical Activity
Sleep
Stress / Emotional Wellbeing / Connectedness
90% reduced risk for heart disease by 50% lower Cholestrol, 6mmHg lower BP, Stop smoking, ideal BMI, >150mins moderate exercise/week, 5 veg + 2 fruit per day, manage your stress.

LOCAL STORIES

I performed a stent procedure on a 63-year-old man who has attended my clinic for years. He takes his medication and I was surprised to find new heart disease that needed a stent within two years. After the procedure we spoke about why this might have happened only for him to admit that he had lapsed on his healthy eating, his weight and physical activity. Many people are like this man, and it just shows how damaging a poor lifestyle can be to heart health despite medication.

I treat a family from the Travelling community in Ireland who have a significant family history of heart disease and premature death of some family members in their thirties. Most members smoke and have very little health literacy, although the mothers and older siblings do know the most. The challenge here is education about heart health and the risk of sudden death, seeking treatment when symptomatic, stopping smoking and heavy drinking, and being active. After that, education and support are continuous, introducing healthy eating and giving these patients access to learning, self-care, cardiac rehabilitation and primary/community care services. At the same time, a simple daily routine-based approach to health can be remarkably successful for changing behaviour.

In contrast, a 55-year-old lady attended for a CT heart scan that was normal (11 years after an abnormal scan), because she had stopped smoking, lowered stress, and changed her diet.

Covid-19 has highlighted poor health habits in the population. Behaviours were either pre-existing or have deteriorated since Covid-19. This increases immediate mortality from Covid-19 or builds a path to chronic disease caused by bad lifestyle health habits. The latter will lead to heart disease, strokes, cancer and premature death.

Covid-19 serves as a useful trigger for behaviour change. In Long Covid illness, psychological factors contribute to recovery. I find that coaching new habits (stopping coffee and alcohol) help recovery.

CAN WE CURE HEART DISEASE?

The *TRANSACTIONAL* treatment includes stents, surgery, medications and cardiac rehabilitation. However, while these interventions may deal with the problem you present with, they alone do not reverse the disease or the root cause of the heart problem. This is mending the issue but we still need ways to fix the underlying cause of the problem. Patients are expected to take the medicine and to practice self-care.

Stents and heart surgery improve survival for patients with heart attacks, for those with all three heart arteries blocked, and for heart failure and diabetes patients, especially among patients with symptoms or if medication is not working.

Most patients with heart disease do not have symptoms and must take tablets to control the disease or combine fewer or no medications with lifestyle behaviour management (under doctor supervision). Many patients do not want to take tablets as it is usually lifelong. Most do not change the root causes of why they get heart disease in the first place.

The *TRANSFORMATION* approach is a combination of education and treating the root cause and presenting issues. This is conventional treatment combined with patient behaviour change (behaviour cardiology).

Historically, drug trials have looked at the effect of taking medications and have not looked at behaviour change as an option or the combination of medication with health behaviour change compared with drug treatment alone. Newer diabetes trials show that the combination of exercise, diet and medication reduced chronic illness, heart disease and achieved sustained weight loss over three years, compared with taking the medication alone and not changing lifestyle behaviours.

Real-world patients are more complex than clinical trials: A patient told me how he monitors his blood sugar and keeps it at elevated levels during his day so that he does not have low sugars causing blackouts during work meetings, even though high sugars are not good for his heart health. The same man is overweight and has options to improve his health (healthy eating, exercise, better sleep) and to avoid his less-than-healthy approach to sugar management. It is important to acknowledge that the everyday environment has an enormous impact on health behaviour.

Heart medications do not treat all the root causes of heart disease, e.g. statins do not treat stress, inactivity or your sleep problems. In some patients, medications may affect activity and sleep to the detriment of their heart health.

4

Physical Health: Prevent, Treat and Reverse Heart Disease

Lifestyle medicine is evidence-based medicine in which comprehensive lifestyle changes are used to prevent, treat and potentially reverse the progression of chronic diseases (like heart disease) by addressing the root causes. Doctors deliver it.

It is the role and responsibility of doctors to coordinate a team of health professionals to deliver on the various aspects of lifestyle. That might include a nutritionist, physiotherapy, a personal trainer, psychologist, and referral to addiction services. General practitioners (GPs) provide preventative care for all health issues and occupational health has a key role in terms of employee health and wellbeing.

Lifestyle medicine promotes doctor self-awareness and self-care. It is evidence based. There are six pillars:

- Physical activity
- Healthy eating
- Stress management
- Sleep management

- Social connection
- Addictions (smoking, drugs, alcohol)

It reduces heart disease, improves length of life and reduces blockages in heart arteries. Healthy eating programmes can reverse Type-2 diabetes, hypertension and high cholesterol.

The DIRECT trial showed that a 12-week programme of weight management (low carbohydrate diet) directed by nutrition coaching led to significant weight loss and reversed diabetes in almost 60 per cent of patients. The DASH diet – enriched in fruit and vegetables, low in fat and cholesterol – reverses hypertension. Plant-based diets reduce inflammation and LDL cholesterol compared with standard diets.

Ornish Lifestyle Medicine and the Complete Health Improvement Programme (CHIP) are multidisciplinary lifestyle medicine programmes that improve cardiac outcomes in heart patients.

EXERCISE AND PHYSICAL ACTIVITY

There is compelling evidence that exercise:

- Prevents weight gain
- Reduces weight when combined with lowered calorie intake
- Improves lung and heart fitness
- Prevents falls
- Reduces depression
- Reduces anxiety
- Boosts cognitive function in the elderly
- Reduces lung and endometrial cancer
- Improves bone density and insulin sensitivity
- Increases sleep quality, work-life balance and daily routine functioning

People who exercise live longer and have less heart disease. Physical activity of at least one hour per week reduces all-cause mortality by 15 to 20 per cent, and reduces diabetes, cardiac, stroke, dementia and cancer risk. Doing 10,000 steps each day reduces risk of heart disease by 47%. Any steps above 3000 per day has a heart health benefit.

Physical activity is medicine. The American Heart Association and European Society of Cardiology recommend exercise of 150 to 300 minutes of moderate physical activity per week at moderate intensity or 75 minutes of vigorous physical activity in bouts of any length or an equivalent combination. Light activity is beneficial even in people who are performing no moderate to vigorous physical activity.

For more extensive health benefits, 300 minutes of moderate intensity physical activity or 150 minutes of vigorous physical activity or an equivalent combination and resistance/muscle strengthening at least twice per week is recommended.

Exercise refers to any movement that works your body at a greater intensity than your usual level of daily activity. Exercise raises your heart rate and works your muscles and is mostly done to achieve the aim of physical fitness.

Cardiac exercise

Exercise includes aerobic cardiovascular, resistance/strength training, flexibility/stretching, posture/balance training. There are structured exercise and lifestyle exercise solutions. Moderate paced exercise is associated with less cancer spread and slower growth of a primary cancer lesion.

Exercise intensity can be prescribed using FITT prescriptions and personalised by the talk/sing test (ability to talk/sing while exercising); or targeted heart rates (227–age = 100 per cent maximum heart rate). The least objective but easiest to measure is the talk test. When performing physical activity at a low intensity an individual should be able to talk or sing while exercising. At a moderate intensity, talking is comfortable but singing, which requires a longer breath, becomes more difficult. At vigorous intensity, neither singing nor prolonged talking is possible. Aerobic activity includes brisk walking, cycling, swimming, dancing, tennis, building up to 15,000 steps per day.

Resistance-based training

Resistance (strength) training is a form of physical activity that is designed to improve muscular fitness by exercising muscles/muscle groups against external resistance. The recommendation is one hour two or three days per week. Resistance-based training:

- Leads to better muscle function, which means fewer falls, better performance and less fatigue
- Reduces osteoporosis and increases bone mineral density by 3 per cent
- Boosts strength
- Improves cholesterol and blood sugar levels
- Reduces body fat
- Is as powerful as cardio exercises at reducing heart disease risk
- Is the cornerstone for healthy ageing and longevity

Resistance training is also important for treating back pain after sitting at a desk for prolonged periods of time, including working from home on a computer.

This training can be done with resistance bands, body weight exercises, push-ups, press-ups, bridges, dumbbells, medicine balls, or heavy work around the home/garden. Resting in between strength training days is important.

Strength training should be heavy enough that you complete eight to twelve repetitions before needing a break. Patients should complete three sets of eight to twelve repetitions with short (one- to four-minute) breaks in between each set. A resistance routine is 30 minutes. It should be prescribed along with aerobic exercise prescriptions and the intensity increases slowly over time.

Balance and play therapy

Balance is a predictor of all-cause mortality. Standing on one leg for ten seconds predicts overall mortality.

Playing and having fun promote physical activity. Fun and emotion drive positive health habits and behaviour changes. Children who play experience less future stress. It is so important to find those ways to step away and restore oneself through fun. This means:

- Enjoyment
- Engagement
- Being active
- Freedom from time constraints
- Less worry or self-consciousness
- Flow
- Happiness

Fun is different for everyone – some like doing puzzles, others like playing in the park or doing art.

Play and having fun:

- Reduces stress
- Improves memory
- Improves concentration
- Creates connection
- Improves sleep

Finding ways to bring fun into your life and to smile every day is the cornerstone of all health behaviour change and finding real purpose. Enjoying the behaviour creates positive health habits and the greatest benefit is to be had by doing things with friends, family and colleagues.

Covid-19 and physical activity

The story of exercise and Covid-19 is interesting – young, fit patients are more at risk of Long Covid illness but less likely to have serious acute Covid-19 outcomes. Unfit, unhealthy patients do worse acutely with risk of premature death.

The role of physical activity as treatment depends on Long Covid patient symptoms:

- If fatigue/exhaustion is a major component then only light exercise is allowed.
- If patients are less tired, then gradual increase in exercise with a 10 per cent increase every 10 days is suggested.
- The most important thing is taking small steps and not an all-or-nothing approach.

This is important as Covid-19 can worsen when patients try to exercise too much (90 per cent experience a post-exertion malaise). This may be due to autonomic dysfunction and its effect on heart rate.

Most Long Covid patients were previously healthy and exercised before they acquired Long Covid. In general, exercise reduces severity of original Covid -19illness. A remarkably similar picture is observed in chronic fatigue syndrome and post-viral illness sufferers.

ADDICTIONS – SMOKING AND ALCOHOL

Stopping smoking reduces the risk of heart disease to that of a non-smoker within two years. It increases wellbeing, libido, longevity and leads to less infections and a decrease in premature ageing.

Reduced alcohol intake has similar health benefits, along with better blood pressure, less atrial fibrillation, stroke risk and metabolic conditions like obesity and diabetes.

Smoking increases lung disease which is a marker for poor outcomes with Covid-19.

EMOTIONAL AND MENTAL HEALTH

Mind-body medicine:

- Uses evidence-based effects of thoughts, beliefs and emotions to positively influence physical health.
- Includes relaxation exercises, meditation, yoga, tai chi, conscious breathing and other methods to promote health and healing.
- The purpose is to provide for both primary and secondary prevention of disease rather than acute illnesses.
- A creative, positive, optimistic and grateful mindset helps patients recover from acute illness.
- Removing stress, fear and limiting beliefs from your mind creates free time and energy to engage in fun healthy purpose-filled living.

Dealing with stress has many approaches, including stress management and resilience training. Lifestyle changes are a key component of resilience, as are:

- Positive psychology
- Mindfulness
- Meditation
- Yoga
- Tai chi

- Box breathing (conscious breathing)
- Eliciting the relaxation response that lowers heart rate and blood pressure with breathing
- Coping skills
- Confidence
- Humour
- Altruism (being generous to others)
- Practising gratitude
- Having strong social skills

Mind-body medicine proposes that your thoughts and beliefs impact on your health. If you catastrophize and worry you tend to be sicker. Changing your mindset helps to prevent illness and disease. In some cases, it can reverse disease. Heart-mind-body connections affect heart health, heart disease risks and outcomes. Optimism, purpose and happiness improve heart health compared with stress, depression and anxiety. The mind-body connection is mediated through inflammation, glucose metabolism, lipids, haemostasis and coagulation that are aggravated by chronic stress.

Managing stress:

- Reduces cardiovascular disease
- Improves blood pressure control
- Improves insomnia
- Reduces lower back pain
- Reduces migraine frequency
- Improves arthritis pain control
- Limits incontinence
- Improves disease management such as cancer treatment tolerance

Positive psychological factors are critical to heart health and represent the foundation behind most risk factors for heart disease. Positive psychology and lifestyle medicine are interrelated.

ROLE OF STRESS IN COVID-19

Stressed individuals are more prone to viral illnesses. Covid-19 itself increases stress and in turn increases risk of more Covid-19 infections.

THE SOCIAL CONNECTION

There are strong evidence-based associations between social ties and health. Isolation increases all causes of mortality by 40 per cent. In the same study from UK Biobank, having more social connections (especially with family) is associated with significantly lower morbidity and mortality. The benefits of social connection are related to:

- Social engagement
- Companionship
- Social control
- Role-based purpose
- Meaning in connection with others
- Self-esteem
- Control
- Belonging
- Less stress

The success of Weight Watchers and Alcoholics Anonymous is built around strong social support. Supportive friends help clients to build self-efficacy and control. Social connection can be improved using coaching programmes, online support and phoning family and friends. Disconnection leads to poor lifestyle behaviours, especially over-eating and drinking alcohol.

Socialisation and group activities in the workplace are an important part of stress management. In many cases employees go outside of work to manage their self-care instead of connecting with their colleagues inside the workplace and working through their wellbeing together.

When people come together, teamwork helps every member of the team to improve their health and that is very empowering and motivating, as well as boosting workplace morale, job satisfaction and productivity by being healthier together.

Social determinants of health include structural determinants and conditions in which people are born, grow, live, work, age and they affect the functioning, health and quality of life of the community. These include economic stability, neighbourhood, environment, education, social and community context, health and health care.

Social initiatives that aim to improve heart health include:

- Wellbeing projects
- Million Hearts
- Faith-based interventions
- Healthy community interventions
- Healthy Ireland initiatives
- Walk with a Doc
- Irish Heart Foundation initiatives
- VHI parkrun

HEALTHY EATING

What you eat affects your health. Diet is the number one cause of poor health worldwide. Unhealthy diets are responsible for:

- 25 per cent of global deaths
- 31 per cent of premature deaths in Europe
- 35 per cent of greenhouse gas emissions

Changing what you eat can:

- Lower weight
- Offset disease risk
- Reverse conditions (such as Type-2 diabetes, coronary artery disease and sleep apnoea)

Studies show that:

- Lower weight and normalising body mass index is associated with reduced risk of heart disease in women
- Healthy eating reduces cancer death by 30 per cent and cardiac death by one-third
- Including all lifestyle factors reduces all-cause mortality by 60 to 82 per cent and increases life expectancy by over ten years

Healthier eating has metabolic benefits for everyone and positively contributes to a lower risk of a heart attack. The PURE trial showed that diets with more vegetables, grains, nuts, fish, fruit, plants and legumes lowered the risk of heart disease and cancer. Plant-based diets significantly lower the risk for developing dementia, reduce blood pressure, inflammation, heart failure and chronic disease. Eating avocado instead of bacon, eggs and butter reduces risk for heart disease by 20 per cent.

Meat consumption is associated with an increase in prevalence of coronary artery disease, chronic kidney disease and incident heart failure. The Mediterranean diet and plant-based diets (lots of vegetables and greens) are associated with fewer heart events, strokes, and cancers. The diet includes fruit, vegetables, fish, less meat, olive oil, 10–12 units of alcohol per week, water, coffee, oatmeal, leafy greens, blueberries, almonds, pistachio nuts, sweet potatoes and tomatoes (antioxidant, anti-inflammatory, vitamins). The PrediMed study of the Mediterranean diet included patients aged 50–80 years with at least three risk factors for heart disease. The diet allows small amounts of dairy, plenty of green vegetables, less red meat, more fish and plants, and reduces all-cause mortality from strokes, heart disease and cancer compared with a standard diet. Poor eating habits like skipping breakfast (usually in people with busy lives and other poor lifestyle habits) were associated with higher risk of adverse outcomes.

This healthy-eating approach is akin to the lifestyle seen in 'Blue Zone' areas of the world where the populations live much longer and are healthier compared with other countries. The Blue Zones include Okinawa in Japan, Sardinia in Italy, Nicoya in Costa Rica, Ikaria in Greece and Loma Linda in California.

The Blue Zone diet includes plenty of vegetables, fruit, beans, water, a small amount of coffee, alcohol, no red meat and plenty of fish. The healthy-eating habits are paired with daily physical activity, strong community spirit and communication, socialising, living a life with purpose and not being stressed.

Most HCPs recommend healthy eating approaches that include small portions of:

- Fruit and vegetables
- Healthy sourced protein
- Legumes
- Whole grains
- Less red meat
- More plants
- Chicken and fish (Europe)
- Meat (Australia)
- Not eating processed foods
- Limiting sugar
- Reducing salt intake to an absolute minimum
- Reducing alcohol intake to a minimum
- Drinking plenty of water
- Adding daily physical exercise as part of the healthy eating plan
- Managing stress
- A good sleep routine

The DASH (Dietary Approaches to Stop Hypertension) diet is recommended to treat or reverse high blood pressure. This emphasises:

- Healthy food choices
- Portion control
- Salt restriction to one teaspoon per day.
- Four–five portions of fruit and vegetables daily
- Six–eight servings of grains (cereal, rice, pasta)
- Avoiding fat, butter, cheese and cream
- Low-fat or fat-free dairy are allowed
- Eating nuts and plenty of protein

In general:
- Low-fat diets reduce risk of heart disease and some cancers.
- Little or no red meat in your diet reduces risk of premature cancers (bowel, stomach and prostate).
- Low sugar and low carbohydrate diets help people lose weight and reverse/prevent diabetes.
- The emphasis is to choose healthy eating habits instead of multiple 'yo-yo' restrictive diets.
- Eating intuitively when hungry, in tiny amounts of healthier foods and eating a balanced diet (half a plate of vegetables, a quarter plate of protein and a quarter plate of whole grains), and eating until you feel 80 per cent full is the cornerstone of Blue Zone populations' health survival.

The Ornish Lifestyle Medicine programme (Lifestyle Heart Trial) adopts a whole-food plant-based diet and has demonstrated reversal of heart artery blockages, improvement in chest pain scores and symptoms, and a reduction in risk.

The programme includes healthy eating, an exercise programme, stress management and an emotional wellbeing programme. The same interventions reduce prostate cancer risk and the progression of Alzheimer's disease, and are associated with a longer lifespan compared with a traditional Western diet.

The EPIC study of 23,000 people who exercised for 3.5 hours/week, did not smoke, ate a healthy diet and kept to a healthy weight, prevented 93 per cent of diabetes, 81 per cent of heart attacks, 50 per cent of strokes and 36 per cent of all cancers. Taking supplements does not have any additional cardiovascular benefit.

Long Covid healthy eating

There is no specific Long Covid recovery diet. However, as Covid-19 is driven by autonomic dysfunction and inflammation, it would be prudent to reduce inflammatory foods (white flour-based foods, fried foods, sugary drinks, processed meats, margarine), sugar, alcohol and coffee consumption, and increase water intake.

The Mediterranean diet has anti-inflammatory benefits. Foods like green leafy vegetables, fatty fish and olive oil suppress pro-inflammatory molecule production and enhance the production of anti-inflammatory ones. The Mediterranean diet is best paired with stress reduction techniques like conscious breathing and mindfulness exercises, along with 150–180 minutes of weekly cardiovascular activities and adequate sleep.

Not smoking, managing obesity, reducing alcohol intake, and having a healthy gut microbiome all share anti-inflammatory benefits as well. Low sugar, low fat and high fibre diets promote better gut health. A DASH diet for hypertension has many of these benefits too.

Meditation, tai chi, yoga, and hanging out with positive-minded friends also reduce inflammation.

SLEEP MEDICINE

Few people realise the importance of sleep for heart health, including doctors who treat people with heart issues. Sleep provides energy to get through each day. Long Covid illness patients with poor sleep struggle to function mentally and physically, and experience profound tiredness. Improving sleep quality and duration improves recovery and wellbeing.

There has been a 60 per cent increase in prevalence of sleep disturbances with Covid-19. This triggers stress, poor wellbeing and depression. This is getting worse as people are always switched on to work too. Many people have developed Covid-related insomnia (Coronosomnia). This comes with inferior quality sleep, more screen time, overeating and nightmares.

Sleep:

- Improves memory and concentration
- Enhances learning and neuroplasticity
- Is cardioprotective
- Soothes emotions and mental fatigue
- Reduces inflammation in the body
- Optimises physiological growth and repair
- Regulates brain activity
- Restores body function

Deep sleep is needed most for daily brain recovery. Effective sleep management:

- Reduces weight gain, heart problems and improves mental/ emotional health.
- The daily recommendation is 6–8 hours (only 50 per cent of the US population get seven hours' sleep).
- 3 percent of the population are short sleep phenotypes who only need under six hours.
- Circadian rhythm affects melatonin, cortisol, body temperature, blood pressure, heart rate, immune response and bone remodelling.

- Sleep deprivation affects safety, attention, fall risk, chronic health, e.g. heart, the immune system, and weight gain increases with less sleep.
- Better sleep reduces heart attack risk.
- Taking a midday 40-minute nap is associated with health improvement.

Obstructive sleep apnoea, Willis Ekbom disease (restless legs) and narcolepsy are pathological conditions that affect sleep. The overweight, high-blood-pressure patient who snores and falls asleep during the day should be assessed for sleep apnoea. Willis Ekbom disease is characterised by restless arm and leg movements induced by rest, worse at night and relieved by physical activity (moving around).

Many poor lifestyle habits such as mobile phone use, late nights, alcohol and excess coffee consumption contribute to poor sleep patterns, as do medical issues such as reflux, chronic pain and medications.

'Sleep hygiene' is the practice of changing these habits. Examples are:

- Keeping to a regular bedtime routine.
- Going to bed at the same time every night.
- Having no mobile phones in the bedroom.
- Getting out of bed if not sleeping and only getting back in when tired.
- A diet with more vegetables, less carbohydrates, smaller portions and regular eating times improves sleep.
- Calming measures such as prayer, reading a poem, practising gratitude, having a schedule/routine, light exercise, blue light and turning off devices all help improve sleep.
- Failing that, cognitive behavioural therapy or short-term medications (such as melatonin) are options.

Sleep management is critical for Long Covid management. Poor sleep quality and duration lead to slow recovery and limit the ability of a patient to function physically and mentally each day. Exhaustion limits exercise capacity and in patients who exercise too much the fatigue will get worse. Sleep can be improved with sleep hygiene measures, adding melatonin and/or sleeping tablets where necessary. Meditation, mindfulness and taking a hot bath may also help. Cognitive behaviour therapy is the cornerstone of treatment for insomnia.

SECTION TWO

Emotional Health

5

Thoughts and Behaviours

The World Health Organization defines 'whole health' as emotional, mental, spiritual and psychological health and not merely the absence of disease. Health is more complex than seeing it only as a disease to be fixed.

People do not take their personal health seriously enough to do something about it until they get sick. Many find excuses to avoid dealing with their health: 'Sure, it will never happen to me', despite having an unhealthy lifestyle.

Advancing age and milestone birthdays like 60 years (if you are alive by that age) frequently trigger a medical check-up with the doctor (of interest, retirement adds a 2 per cent annual increased risk of male death over 62 years of age) and a first opportunity for many to see objectively how unhealthy they are.

The limiting step to taking care of health is FEAR! Fear of missing living life, rather than the fear of getting heart disease or dying prematurely. Fear of having to change your status quo. Over 90 per cent of people make no real effort to change their life; they find ways not to make any change.

Women have an advantage if they are attending for cervical smears, breast checks or if they are having babies as each of these times represents an opportunity to check in on their health. Women tend to talk to each other about health issues and will do something about their own concerns. Men tend not to share such concerns with each other. It is only when a friend takes ill/dies that men will be most triggered to visit their doctor.

These situations may lead to a referral for heart tests and seeing a cardiologist, or being given clear advice to watch diet, stop smoking and take up exercise – all excellent and appropriate strategies, sadly ignored by many patients. In fairness to patients, however, everyone has a short attention span and anyone can forget what the doctor has told them.

Time in a doctor's office is usually short and may be rushed. Many patients are afraid and distracted coming to see a doctor. They misplace written information and several go to social media or a friend to find their trusted health information, reassuring themselves that: 'I am fine so there is nothing to worry about.'

We are all afraid of missing out, changing things and we just want to live and let live. Sometimes that choice leads to heart disease and premature death, cancer, Alzheimer's, mental illness and preventable accidents.

Very few unhealthy people will live long lives and those who do may suffer life-long disability, such as paralysis caused by a stroke. There is a need to change fear into a more positive empowering call to be healthy each day and live a long healthy life.

Fear of dying does not seem to alarm enough people (probably because as humans we cannot reason it) but fear of a disabling chronic disease such as Alzheimer's, or the cost of living with a life-long sickness or stroke, does scare people: 'I don't want that, what can I do to prevent that?' they say. There are blood thinners that can reduce stroke risk but not eliminate it. The only cure is prevention.

HEALTH BEHAVIOUR MODELLING

The Health Behaviour Model shows that our health behaviour is defined by four central factors:

- Perceived susceptibility to a condition
- Perceived severity of that condition
- Perceived benefits of behaviour/lifestyle change
- Perceived barriers to making that change

Unfortunately, most people only see barriers. They know what is unhealthy but choose not to change. A few patients don't have any health literacy or know how to change behaviour. Patients must take responsibility for health and be part of their own solution. One saying I like is, 'I cannot do the press-ups for them.'

The Dalai Lama was once asked what surprised him most about humanity. He answered:

'Man, because he sacrifices his health in order to make money; then he sacrifices money to recuperate his health and then he is so anxious about the future that he does not enjoy the present, the result being that he does not live in the present or the future, he lives as if he is never going to die and then dies having never really lived.'

Denial of having a health problem is a major reason for illness and the huge financial cost of treating it. Real wealth comes from being in good health. In fact, good health will make you money. As the saying goes, 'Health is the first million euros that you earn in life.' Sadly, many people believe that having lots of money is the only way to become healthy and happy. Also, people often choose to deny any health problem exists (believing 'it will never happen to me'), and time goes by, only for many people to reach retirement with regrets for not having looked after their health better.

Bronnie Ware, a hospice care nurse in Australia, penned a book based on questions she asked dying patients about their lives. Their greatest regrets were:

- Working all the time and not having the courage to live a life true to themselves
- Wishing that they had not worked so hard (they missed their kids growing up and their partner's companionship by spending so much time on the treadmill of work)
- Wishing that they had the courage to express their feelings (many developed illnesses relating to bitterness and resentment for not becoming who they were truly capable of becoming)
- Wishing that they had stayed in touch with their friends (losing out through overwork and not making enough time or effort); as a result, they experienced loneliness in illness/death
- Wishing that they had let themselves be happier (happiness is a choice: we can sometimes become stuck in the comfort of familiarity and in our emotions and physical lives). Fear of change made them pretend to others and themselves that they were content when deep within they longed to laugh properly and have silliness in their life again.

It is only when the cost to human life is high enough (serious illness, usually) that most people make a health change, but many leave that too late in life when cancer or heart disease have set in or spread beyond the point of curative treatment.

6

Love Your Heart and
Be Grateful to Be Healthy

Despite huge efforts to save patients' lives and giving many a second chance at life, people come back with the same stories of more symptoms, don't want to stay on medications and want to move on with life as if a stent has cured them and act as though having a heart attack is no big deal. Some do not come back at all.

It is amazing what some people take for granted when it comes to dealing with why they developed a life-threatening heart problem in the first place. Many people in the 40–70-year-old age group live remarkably busy lives of consumption: a life of must-have-all, long hours of work, less pleasure, more money, holidays and job promotions. Many are workaholics, burned out, under pressure, stressed, unhappy and cannot stop living this way, primarily because they cannot take the time to stop and see what is going on.

Several have a victim mindset, where they believe that the events of life are responsible for their circumstances, and they are not responsible for their health. 'That is the doctor's job, not mine!' 'This is a disease and not due to my lifestyle choices.' This mindset is common in growing numbers of heart patients compared to those patients who take responsibility and commit to improving their health.

It is curious when asking thriving 80-year-old patients what is so different for them compared to the younger generation of patients like their own children?

They point to their children's lives of:

- Mobile phones
- An always-on, non-stop life
- Higher stress levels
- Longer work hours
- Relationships
- Spiritual health
- Challenging financial circumstances: cost of living and housing
- Overconsumption and not having enough in life
- A fear of missing out on what others have, often driven by social media
- Not being happy and healthy or allowing life to flow and flourish

I returned to Ireland from working as a cardiologist in the United States in 2007. This was a milestone in disruptive technology. Smartphones and social media were launched here soon after my return and cardiology practice took on an entirely new context to what I had trained in.

The new technology was fantastic for easy access to useful information but with time it has created umpteen heart health issues, fear of missing out, the demands for instant gratification, a must-have-everything-and-more-now attitude, unregulated fake online health care advice, and increased risk of heart attacks based on social media platform user behaviours.

Empowering heart patients to practice self-care, take medication, stop smoking, eat better and exercise can save lives.

- A study of heart attack patients in Ireland shows that over 50 per cent do not take their medications or make lifestyle changes to prevent problems, even having had a heart attack and knowing the risk of having another one or even sudden death.
- 90 per cent of heart bypass surgery patients in the United States have not changed their health behaviours and lifestyle at two years after surgery.
- 10 per cent of Irish cancer patients continue to smoke after their lung cancer diagnosis. Even more heart attack smokers do the same.
- Only 8 per cent of people stick to their New Year's health resolutions like stopping smoking, losing weight, reducing alcohol and getting better work-life balance, as examples.
- In the United States only 3 per cent of the population eat a healthy diet.
- 20 per cent of Ireland's population are awaiting hospital medical appointments for chronic diseases caused by lifestyle choices and social circumstances.
- Ireland is also set to become one of the most obese countries in Europe.

However, all is not lost: there are real reasons to be grateful for medical practice, its science and treatments. From the early days of Hippocrates, founder of medicine, to modern-day Nobel laureates, simple steps, ideally learned and practiced from birth to grave, make the greatest impact on personal health.

BEHAVIOUR CARDIOLOGY

I empower the whole patient (mind, heart and body). This includes their purpose and attitude, and how that aligns with their health goals. This engages physical, emotional, and behavioural health and improves outcomes. It empowers the patient, their family and community to find ways that make everyone's health a priority and to undertake positive healthy behaviours each day.

People fail to realise how short their life is (20–30,000 days from birth), especially when 30 per cent is spent sleeping, 60 per cent working and 10 per cent on everything else. For many readers, you may already have used up 10,000–15,000 days!

I have trained as a cardiologist, lifestyle medicine and mind-body physician, and as a health habits coach, and I have acquired skills to help patients design ways that transform their health habits.

I do my best to be healthy each day. I set daily health intentions. I complete small healthy personal and professional behaviours that align with my health goals. I know (based on scientific evidence) that if I am seen to look after my health, 80 per cent of my patients will follow this example. Several colleagues have shared how their patients stopped smoking after learning their doctor had done the same.

I fully understand that heart health is not a simple matter (nor is any area of medicine). Life is affected by many factors, including financial, spiritual, emotional, mental, professional, personal, educational and health. All of these are inter-related: as an example, your financial circumstances may influence physical health, eating options, work obligations and mental health at the same time. Giving you mood tablets for mental health concerns does not solve your financial or work issues. How you think and respond to the events of your life determine what outcomes you will achieve.

HUMAN FACTORS: SNIPER'S ALLEY

Every day I meet colleagues and friends who share stories about someone they know with new significant heart problems. Many of these patients are fit and healthy, usually cyclists or runners, with no known heart-risk factors. Many have high-powered jobs, such as the story of a 58-year-old friend who collapsed and was resuscitated by a passerby who happened to be a doctor; he was shocked fifteen times and transferred alive to hospital, only to discover he had a blocked artery and had a stent placed in his main coronary artery.

A similar story is that of a 57-year-old man who collapsed on a treadmill in a gym and was successfully resuscitated with fourteen shocks by a doctor who happened to be exercising nearby and was able to get a defibrillator and save him. This man was a smoker and ended up with a lifesaving stent in the same main artery and an implanted cardiac defibrillator. Another colleague, aged in his late fifties, collapsed at work, was rushed into the cardiac unit and had a stent placed in his main coronary artery. He was usually well but admitted to having a stressful job as well as poor drinking and eating habits.

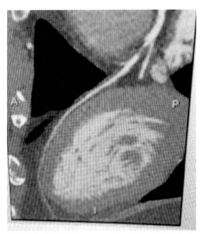

• CT OF LAD NARROWING

CT of LAD narrowing

A dear medical friend was 'feeling a bit off, but [it's] nothing worrying'. He was 58 years old too, a non-smoker, a little over-weight, had a terribly busy medical job but took regular time off. However, he always seemed to be rushing. 'Feeling a little unwell' became chest pain and he ended up in hospital. He had a cardiac arrest and did not survive.

The list goes on and on. But it is not just men; women get stressed at work and in life, but in fairness many women will present earlier to hospital and get assessed. The challenge can be their symptoms may be atypical and a heart diagnosis may be missed. But the truth in all these cases lies in risk factors. Why do we have this cluster of near-fatal heart attacks in fit people, and doctors burning out only to have similar near-fatal, and unfortunately sometimes fatal, heart events too?

Being fit does not stop heart attacks if the same person has other life issues, like mounting chronic stress. Many people believe that a weekend run or cycle will fix their stress problems. Dealing with the underlying root of the problem is the only way to resolve stress issues. Procrastination is likely to run a risk for similar cardiac events. If you are struggling with stress, then getting checked out by a doctor and preventing these problems is the only solution. Given the risks for heart disease, a cardiology assessment is essential.

THE COVID FACTOR FOR PATIENTS

Emotional health issues have exploded since the Covid-19 pandemic: people cocooned at home with no family nearby, they were not exercising outside, could not even go to church, were not meeting other people; they are stressed out, leading to physical and often heart health problems. Add to that war, inflation and financial crises, and the constant 'doom and gloom' in the media every day and it leads to more health problems.

People start to complicate their life by negative thinking, rumination and catastrophizing. In heart health this mindset can cause symptoms, anxiety and make people sick or seriously ill. Lifting Covid restrictions has helped people deal with their thoughts and beliefs in a more positive way, partly due to meeting up with friends and family. It is important for people to remember that 'you did not cause the Covid-19 pandemic, it happened, and you are not responsible for its consequences'. You are responsible for how you respond to it and that defines your situation including your health. 'You can choose your health or hold on to the past and procrastinate.'

Connecting Emotional and Physical Heart Health

7

My Whole Heart Health Model

My Whole Heart Health approach:

- Is designed for a balanced, purposeful way of living
- Addresses physical, behavioural and lifestyle heart health (including emotional health), and social health connection (mind, heart, and body)

Patients are assessed for heart disease, and undergo tests to look at their heart pump, blood vessels and the electrical system. All this information, along with blood results, are analysed to decide if/what medications need to be prescribed and if stents or surgery are required, and plan for that process

Part Two of the assessment is to understand the root cause of the heart problems, the patient's health behaviours, their thoughts and emotions, and desire to change.

I then design a personalized balanced lifestyle plan that addresses these factors.

WHOLE HEALTH MODEL VALIDATION

The Whole Health Model has been validated by colleagues in the United States. The Veterans Administration (VA) hospitals and the Whole Health Institute have designed a purpose-focused approach to general health care, aligned by equipping patients with physical and emotional health interventions, clinical care and connecting with community, work and social supports.

Whole Health USA empowers and equips people to take charge of their physical, mental and spiritual health. It comprises seven principles:

1. Self-awareness: what is my health like now and where am I trying to get to?
2. Discovering life's purpose (living a full and meaningful life): starting from purpose, joy is what matters most even during suffering. This becomes the foundation of health and self-care.
3. Capacity to heal from the inside: comes from body and mind, self-care and optimising both.
4. Holism: Treating the whole patient rather than symptoms of disease.
5. Power of experience: brings inner peace, joy, passion, hope and a connection with what could be.
6. Skill building: finding a place to learn, practice and to have fun.
7. Support: through connection and belonging. Interconnection brings it all together.

This approach asks the patient 'how do I change the conversation around my future health?'

The purpose of whole health is aligned with:

- Patient health
- The environment
- The community where you live and work

It aspires to 'imagining a day when people's sense of meaning and purpose, their mutuality, interdependence, compassion, and awareness of a collective humanity is profoundly altered'.

This leads to complete physical and emotional health when aligned with physical, behavioural and lifestyle health and is embedded in every community.

My Whole Heart Health is grounded on this framework and possibility for everyone.

<u>My Whole Heart Health starter steps</u>

1. EAT – less sugar, two fruit, five veg each day, grains, less fat, more water, plants, fast 16:8.
2. EXERCISE – Walk 30 minutes each day, stand on single leg for 10 seconds, 10,000 steps.
3. SLEEP – 7 hours each night, early to bed, phone off, cool room temperature.
4. STRESS – gratitude habit, meditate and be positive.
5. SOCIAL – make and meet friends.
6. PURPOSE – do what you love and have fun doing it every moment of every day.
7. CONNECTION – Community, Social determinants of health, Link with GP services.

WHOLE HEART HEALTH – SOCIAL CONNECTION AND TEAM-BASED SUPPORT

The role of community cannot be understated in heart and chronic disease management. Local initiatives such as the HSE Connected Island (or Connected Society UK) have identified ways to prescribe social solutions for patients such as connection with other people.

Other examples are:

• Men's Sheds
• Alone charity

- Irish Farmers Association
- Royal Mail, UK

It is important to go beyond traditional locations (outside clinical settings) to places where people live, learn, work, play and pray within neighbourhoods and communities. Considering the social and cultural context of individuals and their families is at the heart of community-based interventions. This also provides feedback to better understand community health needs.

Raising awareness of the social determinants of health include:

- Providing community resources
- Building a support networks of friends
- Meeting places
- Volunteering opportunities to help people. Opportunities to call on them or visit for a cup of tea, go for a walk – these are some practical steps and are all available for free in Ireland.
- Recognising people who are lonely or isolated, listening and communicating with them through their stories helps to improve their health and wellbeing.

It is so important for children to use the community to foster their own resilience and self-nurture. This might be by playing sport at a local club or acting as a buddy/support to an elderly neighbour or doing newspaper delivery rounds.

International health projects such as TILDA (The Irish Longitudinal Study on Ageing) or the Blue Zones Longevity population show the importance of tribe and living with like-minded people as initiative-taking ways to boost health habits. The close communities of Blue Zone areas live longer.

In TILDA studies of people above 60 years of age living in Ireland, isolation and loneliness increase morbidity and mortality. This is seen more so in lower socioeconomic and unhealthy population groups. These people also had the highest burden of death during Covid-19, both here in Ireland and around the world.

Studies of the Mediterranean diet also highlight the power of social connection and community in addition to diet and exercise as a predictor of improved heart health. Social prescribing initiatives of group activities, physical activity and living supports have all been shown to improve health. Simple practices such as hugging, saying 'hello' and 'thank you', altruism and random acts of kindness, gratitude and compassion go a long way towards helping people's health. Promoting behaviours that physically connect people with fun in mind are ideal.

CARDIAC REHABILITATION PROGRAMMES

Existing cardiac rehabilitation programmes show consistent and significant health gains with a group-based Intensive Lifestyle Management approach. However, they are provided after a cardiac event has occurred and not before. Programmes in the United States, such as the Ornish Heart Disease Reversal and CHIP programmes, provide similar heart patients with an intensive rehabilitation offering that includes nutrition, exercise, self-love, relationships and social connection lifestyle pillars to manage and even undo heart disease.

In Ireland, we provide cardiac rehabilitation for heart patients after heart attacks, stents, or surgery. These programmes run for six weeks and help to kickstart patients into heart disease awareness, exercises, insights on medications and the need to eat and live a healthier life.

These programmes motivate patients to improve their heart health using information and exercises over the six weeks and encourage them to join and follow a community exercise programme (usually at free or low cost), but 50 per cent of patients tend to take matters into their own hands at six weeks and go back to their usual pre-heart event routine at home.

Technology-driven virtual rehabilitation programmes allow longer follow-up and have greater positive lifestyle behaviour impact after three months. It is likely that supervised follow-up is what drives the sustained behaviour change. This suggests that most patients require long-term handholding to help change their health behaviours.

Rehabilitation programmes are now in place to help patients recovering from Covid-19 or with Long Covid illness. At our hospital, these programmes have a multidisciplinary team including physiotherapy, occupational therapy, clinical psychology, consultant respiratory and cardiology inputs. Like in cardiac rehabilitation, patients undergo a series of exercise routines and breathing exercises; receive medication advice and return-to-work advice; and focus on symptoms such as sleeping issues, brain fog, and heart and lung symptoms, some of which require medication to support their recovery.

However, resources are limited to provide specialised rehabilitation programmes for an entire population. It is the patients' choice whether they look after their personal health or not, including taking medical advice, following up by attending at clinics, seeing the doctor, taking medications and changing their unhealthy habits.

WHOLE HEART HEALTH COACHING

The Whole Heart Health approach is a game-changer: patients discover their true purpose in self-awareness; they transform their behaviour with support and coaching. These interventions reduce heart disease progression and plaque in arteries, and reverse related risk factors like diabetes, high blood pressure and cholesterol.

This is preventative cardiology which has existed for over 30 years, but many patients have not followed the advice. The greatest opportunity for real prevention is to change the way of living so that people defer heart disease until late in lifespan, without any risk of premature sudden death.

This transformation-led approach:

- Helps patients to help themselves
- Builds motivation, confidence and engagement
- Relies on patient self-awareness and insights (the more you see, the more you can intentionally make changes)
- Strives to help patients find their own answers
- Focuses on what is working well
- Encourages collaboration

Coaches display an unconditional positive regard for their clients and a belief in their capacity for change, honouring the fact that each client is an expert on their own life, while ensuring that all interactions are respectful and non-judgmental.

Health coaching is well studied and there are reports of improvements in diet self-management, reduction in diabetes, reduced stress and higher satisfaction with self-care. In asthma it reduces repeat hospitalisations and in cancer patients the approach is known to improve pain severity compared with standard doctor care.

There are hundreds of clinical coaching papers. All report significant improvement in lifestyle factors, wellbeing and quality of life in COPD patients, as well as in diabetes. Longer duration of coaching results in better blood sugar control in diabetes. The latter approach includes setting goals, education, individualised care and frequent follow-up. A review of 284 coaching papers summarised the most effective approaches used. This identified a patient-centred approach, patient-determined goals, self-discovery and active learning, accountability for behaviours, education and consistent ongoing relationship.

The COACH Program in Australia includes patients with diagnosed heart disease who underwent cardiac rehabilitation and coaching. These patients achieve significant sustained improvements in cholesterol levels, smoking cessation, healthy eating and activity. Follow-up calls at two years showed consistent healthy weight control, regular physical activity, achieving target blood pressure control, cholesterol levels and lower hospital use compared with patients who were not coached. At a six-year follow-up, this translated to 5 per cent reduction in all-cause deaths, especially among men who received more than four coaching sessions. This programme is available throughout Australia.

Coaching is a collaboration between the doctor and patient, starting with empathy, aligned with motivation, growing confidence, creating SMART (Specific, Measurable, Achievable, Relevant, Time-Based) goals and setting accountability. It works best by keeping it simple and easy for people to make changes, so they feel great about doing and want to do more, like exercising, and it is about meeting patients where they are at, instead of starting all over again.

These prevention opportunities also apply to cancer, mental illnesses, Alzheimer's disease and lung diseases. Patients must set clear health intentions/outcomes that focus the effort on improving health (better health to reverse obesity or diabetes for example) and completing SMART goals (like losing twelve pounds weight in six weeks by eating more vegetables and less sugar) or aspirations.

Stories of patient success

A 63-year-old patient attends my clinic with heart risk of high blood pressure and cholesterol. He was 'feeling sluggish, fatigued, breathless and fed up, wanted a better life – tried every diet and always relapsed'. Unexpectedly, he decided that making daily healthy eating choices made sense.

He started immediately and worked on that each day – choosing green vegetables over potatoes; water over wine; cut out sugar; found substitute healthy treats like a square of dark chocolate instead of ice cream after dinner. He did the food shopping. He walked and reduced weight by 28 lbs in seven months.

He feels better than he ever did. He came off cholesterol and blood pressure tablets. His heart health is excellent at present – in fact, his blood pressure and cholesterol levels are now normal, and he is off all medications. He finds that his healthy eating way works for him, and he is sticking with it.

Interestingly, his wife has put on weight and he comments that she has not found her *why* yet, despite seeing his progress.

So, it is not just about wanting to do something and repeating the same actions each day

- There must be a '*why?*' – a real burning desire for change
- *What* do I need to do?
- Do I have a concise strategy to make it work (healthy food choices, doing shopping, starting small and taking your time)
- Setting Daily SMART goals – his vision was being healthier and energetic

My patient chose the SMART goal of losing 28 lbs weight in 28 weeks by eating greens, fruit, smaller portions and no white foods for each meal, every day.

- He started keeping a food diary of his usual weekly eating routines, including what types of food he had, quantities, and when he ate; his water intake; and alcohol consumption.
- He made changes to his food habits, substituting healthy alternatives like salads instead of potatoes; brown foods instead of white; more water and less alcohol.
- He got creative and tried cooking meals and varying foods as an experiment to find healthy habits.
- He had fun in his new culinary routine, which encouraged him to keep doing it.

- Every day he kept his healthy vision alive, took daily steps to eat healthier, celebrated his progress and continued achieving his goal.

New medical treatments for obesity include Semaglutide and Tirazepitide. These injections help patients to lose weight, but they only work if patients change their diet and exercise on the medication. The course of treatment is lifelong.

Stories from these patients are fascinating. Suddenly patients can see exactly where their lifestyle was failing them before. A consequence of this medication is that it causes nausea and that puts people off food and substantial amounts of alcohol. Many will lose weight, reverse diabetes, improve blood pressure and cholesterol levels, and lower their risk of chronic disease. It is not for everyone nor is it first-line, which should be lifestyle- and behaviour-driven.

I have patients who want higher doses of medication only for me to discover that they are not taking behaviour steps seriously and the drug is not working as they are still overeating. Several report that 'they have found ways to eat and drink the same way and take the injection!' Interestingly, three years on from treatment with these drugs, at least half of US patients have stopped taking them and have regained most weight

I share the example of statins and aspirin medicine not being able to treat sleep, stress or physical inactivity. Similarly, blood pressure medicines do not work unless you change lifestyle. Patients want instant gratification and immediate solutions to reverse illness.

There is no instant fix for chronic heart problems, but there is a process to prevent, manage and potentially reverse chronic diseases through lifestyle changes and medication where medically indicated. Ironically, most patients do not want lifelong medication and are not able to make sustained lifestyle changes instead.

Long Covid patients can also benefit from behaviour change interventions, especially for energy, sleep, sleep recovery, activity, psychology/stress and eating lifestyle pillars. These steps do improve Long Covid recovery.

Designing for successful Whole Heart Health behaviour change

New healthy behaviours must:

- Align with your intended goals and vision
- Be easy to do
- Be something that you want to do
- Create a feeling of success. Doing the new behaviour needs to make you feel successful – as you do it you get nearer to achieving the goal.
- Encourage you to repeat the behaviour on each subsequent day
- Drive habits and recovery: emotions do this. Celebrate immediately (smile) as you do the behaviour.
- Instil gratitude, optimism and a positive mental attitude – all of which improve heart health

In order to be successful you should:

- Start with *one* small step (such as adding a single piece of fruit to each meal) and build up (two pieces of fruit). This is the most effective way to achieve long-lasting behaviour change.
- Try not to take on too much at once. Trying to take on board more than two tasks at the same time is doomed to failure.
- Slowly build a new health routine from day one and attempt to do it each day.
- Get the process right instead of building up too quickly. Moving too fast and trying too hard can lead to loss of interest.

- Commit to making the changes immediately. Do not say you will do something and then do nothing at all.
- Accept that progress varies from person to person.
- Remind yourself that you are on a health journey and are not trying to reach a weight loss diet destination.

People will often say to me in the clinic: 'Doctor, I will think about what you said and see.' Usually, the thinking stops the minute they leave the clinic. In other circumstances I will refer them to an exercise trainer or a nutritionist and find out they do not show up or that they find excuses such as the cost being too expensive, rather than considering the cost of doing nothing for their health.

Heart health does not allow for the luxury of waiting until you have a heart attack and attending the exercise programme if you are still alive or able to exercise afterwards. In many cases, patients will look back at previous clinic visits and say, 'Why did I not make the changes last year when we talked about that?'

The critical success factors for permanent health behaviour change are:

- Having a clear focus on being healthier
- Having a goal and being intentional with your behaviours each day to achieve that goal
- Focusing on one day at a time instead of chasing a target is the best way to improve
- Keeping a record of daily progress (by writing it down in a journal, reading and reviewing it every day)

Patients do best if they start where they are at, e.g. if you already exercise, start with that habit first, get the small steps right and then add more health behaviours slowly. Remember that you will not perfect long-lasting behaviour change in one day. You will meet bumps on the road, but faith and persistence will help you reach your goals, even when you feel like giving up. It will require micro-managing, learning what works best, when, where and how for you.

Everyone will have good and bad days, but you need to tweak and commit to doing this every day no matter what. As you move forward, build a routine and you will achieve big rewards for your health. Be open to learning and to iteration. Keep your focus on the goal you are trying to achieve and feel how great it is having achieved that goal now. Hold onto that feeling of achievement every day until your goal is manifested.

One of my patients keeps a little black book and writes down each action he takes for his health every day. He writes everything and reads it each night; he sets to-do tasks every day and swears by this. He shared with me that it helps his self-awareness and daily decisions as to what works and does not work when it comes to eating healthier.

When he is tired, he observes that he eats more and sleeps less. These behaviours will increase his body weight and become a vicious circle. With his black book he told me how he can plan his day, work on behaviours that make the day less tiring and reduce his fatigue so that he does not compensate with emotional eating.

Reversing heart disease and risk factors is possible. The following are helpful:

- Having a vision for your health (vision board can help)
- Redesigning and changing unhealthy behaviours and habits into a healthy daily routine.
- Having a health coach (your doctor) to teach you how to do this.
- Asking friends to keep you accountable and to give regular feedback..

I have helped patients to stop smoking and as they have progressed, I have added behaviours that help improve healthy eating habits so they do not gain weight by eating unhealthy foods instead of smoking, and I have prompted them to take this opportunity to do some walking and grow their physical activity habits.

Long Covid athletes' behaviours

I treat several athlete patients with Long Covid illness who have heart symptoms, some with heart damage, who are keen to return to physical activity. In some cases, these individuals are established international athletes and Covid-19 may decondition them. There are guidelines to help them return to training, but they now require medical supervision. Professional athletes with Covid-19 symptoms must see cardiologists for cardiac and pulmonary testing and then undergo gradual return to sport based on findings.

In many of these cases, I work with sports medicine to help patients achieve that. Many of my usual non-Covid-19 patients who like exercise are also helped in similar ways by medically supervised personalised exercise programmes, which may be based on tailoring heart rates to exercise or diet management and other lifestyle factors. Athletes are interesting patients because when they are very fit and not performing optimally, this may highlight a medical issue, but that might be a non-medical problem. Covid-19 and other viral infections can be one cause, as can diet, sleep, stress, training routine, over-exercising and other illnesses.

These patients come back to the cardiologist/doctor to coordinate the health plan, measure progress and make healthy changes together. In this way patients have the best opportunity to optimise their health and wellbeing in a structured, supported, safe and effective way.

Ironically, behavioural change studies in health care consistently show that having the doctor involved improves the patient commitment and success with sustained change when compared with no coaching at all.

Kickstart Long Covid Recovery – no clear evidence-based practice

- Lifestyle Changes
- Exercise limited by patient's ability, so it must be tailored individually.
- Breathing training
- Sleep Hygine
- Stree Recovery
- Medications if very symptomatic – arrhythmias, palpitations (Procoralan), Stress (TCAs) Sleep (Melatonin) Brain Fog (SSRIs, Naltrexone), Modafinil, Methylphenidate
- Specialist treatment for other problems – ear / balance; GI
- Occupational Health for brain fog, executive function, concentration problems
- Speech Therapy
- Specialised Physiotherapy
- Ongoing International Research groups: NIH Recover Initiative; Ireland Long Covid Research Group; Long Covid Research Consortium

8

What Is Stopping Change?

People struggle to change their lifestyle behaviours and habits. Over 90 per cent think about it or put it off and never change. The real problem lies inside the human mind. What you think and believe determines how you behave and what your habits are. You can choose to close your mind, or you can change your beliefs and behaviours to serve positive health outcomes.

The more often you perform an action or behave in a certain way – visualise having already achieved your health goal and how that makes you feel each day, affirm positive words about your new self, often best said with gratitude ('I am so happy and grateful now that I am eating healthy every day, I live in a healthy body', for example), and share emotions of happiness and gratitude – the more that gets wired into your brain and subconscious mind. Many of my patients practice this each morning to powerful effect.

Your brain can change its physical structure and function based on suggestions from your imagination, behaviours, emotions and thoughts. Your brain can keep changing until the day you die. This

76

is called neuroplasticity. Interestingly, your unconscious mind is unable to tell the difference between real and unreal thoughts.

Making or breaking habits causes neuroplastic changes in your brain. This is supported by dopamine release which reinforces behaviour change and new habits.

If you want to change health habits, then you must:

- Consciously think about how your life would improve by changing your health behaviour. What would that look and feel like? Imagine what that new healthy life would be and feel like for you? Build your desire to be your healthiest best self.
- Go to a room where you will not be disturbed; sit down and close your eyes. Focus your imagination on your desired health goal and what date you will achieve it by (for example losing 14 pounds of weight in 30 days). Keep holding those thoughts intact until you can see them. Trust and have faith in the process and keep feeling that feeling of having your wish fulfilled (you feel great, clothes feel comfortable, you are more energetic and happy). See yourself as being in best health now. Write this out every day, read it and feel it.
- Remind yourself and motivate change with affirmations, visualisations and positive self-talk
- Use your imagination to come up with practical plans to deliver your health goals. Begin at once to see yourself as healthy, demanding and expecting health habit suggestions to come to you. Act on these immediately.
- Put your new action steps to work and build your new healthy habits. Just do it. Don't rely on reason. See yourself doing these steps (exercise, sleep, healthy eating) in return for your best health.
- Celebrate and get support from others to grow new habits.
- Develop new neural pathways through constant repetition and relaxation.
- Cultivate awareness.

- Willpower boosts serotonin release (as does sunlight, exercise and happiness)

Dr Thurman Fleet (1895) discovered ways of healing back problems by planting ideas in the patient's subconscious mind, 'like planting new flowers in a garden originally full of weeds'. His ground-breaking clinical studies formed the basis of what is now Whole Health. He treated patients with a combination of mind and body medical practices referred to as Concept Therapy. This applied a mind-body medicine approach like my Mind Heart Body approach for heart health.

The principles are based as follows:

- Your mind is composed of a conscious and subconscious mind. The former is responsible for 10 per cent of brain activity.

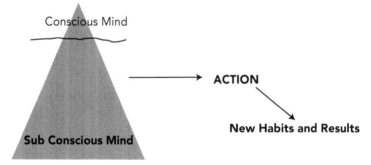

The conscious and subconscious mind

- The conscious mind evolves from birth and informs your behaviour. It receives inputs from the five senses (smell, taste, sight, hearing and touch). It is created from your logic and reason (such as solving maths problems or reasoning different people's opinions). What you learn from books, school, family, parents and friends, and the world around you is absorbed into the conscious mind. You impress your thoughts, feelings and beliefs onto your subconscious mind or else they stay in your conscious mind. The latter effectively guards your subconscious mind. You filter what goes to your subconscious mind using auto suggestions and that helps you to form your new health habits.

- You desire to be your healthy best self and you believe in that. This lifts your energy level. You suggest to the subconscious mind to act on this feeling.

- Your thoughts influence your results. They can be positive ('I can') or negative ('I cannot'), or you can change the latter to 'I can do'. The more you move in a positive can-do direction, the better you feel and that will bring you closer to achieving your goal. This part of your mind is illogical, always switched on day and night, works fast and records everything. It is the feeling mind and is responsible for 90 per cent of your actions.

- It is not enough to wish you are healthy without feeling it. You can blow out your birthday cake candles and setting a goal, writing it down and believing in it make that wish but without taking action, nothing will change. You must hold onto the feeling of achieving your goal to succeed.

- Repetition is key. Gratitude, optimism, visualising and positive affirmations when practiced every day will activate your subconscious mind.

- Interestingly, those positive feelings improve heart health and behaviours. Eliciting positive feelings when doing healthy habits leads to more sustained behaviour change compared with the traditional doctor model of just telling patients about heart risk. Mindset coaching helps patients to sustain healthy eating and regular exercise habits.

- Try doing this for the next 30 days – imagine your healthy best self. Build your desire to be that person. Create a big health goal. Get into the habit of focusing on your health goal, practising gratitude, doing visualisation, affirmations and keeping your desire and emotions burning to be your healthiest self. Keep at this every day until you achieve your goal.

- You need to get into the habit of doing health behaviours to achieve results. Activating your subconscious everyday is half of the process, the other half is taking action: doing behaviours such as eating healthier, drinking water, taking exercise.

Start with one or two behaviours each day, do them immediately as you wake up (gratitude and visualising) and throughout the day (eating less, walking and drinking water). Once you are happy with two, increase to five behaviours each day. Be creative. Make sure the behaviours are easy and enjoyable, so you build more sustainable healthy habits. Keep a written record of how you are progressing and review it each day. Trust in yourself, have faith and always focus on your desired goal.

HEALTHY MINDSET

If you are not in the right frame of mind you will never change your health behaviours and that increases your risk for more health problems, and if you have Long Covid it will slow down your recovery.

Carol Dweck wrote about having a fixed or growth mindset. Most people have both so everyone has the mind to get better. It is just a question of what you choose. Mindset varies depending on the situation. There can be a catastrophic event like a near fatal heart attack or it may be a moment of reality that pushes you to do something about your health.

Having a major acute heart event such as a heart attack, compared to living an unhealthy lifestyle with risks of problems like diabetes/blood pressure, will trigger different psychological responses. The acute major event may well trigger a grief reaction of anger, denial and eventual acceptance. But this may not be enough to trigger patients to amend their health behaviours. It is frustrating as a doctor (when you want to help people) to see this and at the same time watching people continue with unhealthy habits without having a trigger in their own mind to make changes!

Mindset will affect both clinical scenarios – you may choose to accept this health concern and do something about it (growth mindset), or you may deny, ignore and struggle with it (fixed mindset). Your mind is great at getting in your way. It is your survival instinct and it likes to oversee your behaviours. How you respond to life circumstances will determine what happens to you.

Optimism and gratitude practices improve heart health. Positive-minded people have better health outcomes, they live longer, have 30–40 per cent lower heart disease and stroke disease risk, especially in women. This mindset allows people to cope better with stress.

A fixed mindset is associated with inherent negative thinking (limiting beliefs) which leads to overgeneralizing, blaming, labelling, catastrophizing, ruminating, all-or-nothing thinking and jumping to conclusions. Your brain likes negativity as part of its survival function.

People love to blame everyone else for their health problems, while others like to blame failures of previous diets, make excuses of being unable to walk, no time, being too busy and similar reasons. Many fail to realise these excuses are based on a story that they have created and choose to live. Most negative thought processes speed up brain decline, increase the risk for dementia, heart disease, poorer health outcomes and reduced quality of life.

HEART-BRAIN CONNECTION

The brain, heart and body are aligned:

- They use the effects of thoughts, beliefs and emotions (feelings) to positively influence physical health.
- Positive psychology, yoga, tai chi and meditation improve heart health.
- Tai chi and the relaxation response benefit blood pressure control, healthy ageing and mobility, and they are being

evaluated as cardiac rehabilitation tools in heart disease patients.

- Mindfulness, tai chi and Qigong promote techniques such as relaxation exercises and meditation that reduce inflammation and promote health and healing.
- Mindfulness reflects an ever-changing factor of consciousness (Buddhism), while awareness refers to a stable and specific state of consciousness becoming more self-aware as you teach your subconscious mind using visualisation and affirmation tools.
- Awareness helps you to observe your life decisions, actions and helps you understand behaviour: see the 'why' behind your 'why' and find your true purpose. That helps you to process, accept thoughts and let go of fears and limiting beliefs. It involves integrated practices of concentration and penetrative insights.
- Mindfulness practices enhance attention and emotion regulation, reduce stress, burnout, chronic pain, anxiety and depression.
- Meditation creates a state of relaxation. These help you to develop greater self-awareness, so you can focus on more positive ways of shaping your behaviour.
- Mind wandering and mindfulness are divergent mental states with opposing effects on cognitive performance and mental health. Wandering is a negative self-reflection of your past and worry for your future that disrupts performance.
- Mindfulness awareness helps you to focus on the present without cognitive or emotional reaction and is associated with improved task performance and reduced stress-related symptoms.

These insights give you focus and an opportunity to add healthier choices to your daily life such as drinking more water or going for a walk. It is also a wonderful way to slow down. Try going to a quiet relaxing room in your mind, usually looking out at the blue sea and white sand, with boats anchored and everything very still, calm and quiet. The room is painted white, with colourful pictures; sit into a comfortable chair and relax in stillness. Go to this room several times each day and at night before going to sleep. This lowers stress, gives focus and allows any distractions to disappear. Practice makes this more therapeutic.

Mind-body medicine provides primary and secondary disease prevention.

- The best example is stress causing disease.
- The brain biology, neurohormones and chemical pathways respond to chronic stress and cause metabolic syndrome diseases, inflammation, heart attacks and stroke.
- Stress resilience (relaxation response, mindfulness, social support, positive psychology, spiritual connectedness, exercise/ mindful exercise, nutrition/low sugar diet/, sleep/healthy habits/creativity) increases mitochondrial reserve capacity and insulin receptor sensitivity, and decreases innate immunity and oxidative stress.

Managing these factors, designing a healthier behaviour routine, and reducing the stress load means less vulnerability to chronic diseases including heart attacks and strokes.

The Relaxation Response (repeated breathing in and out for few seconds, which creates a calm and relaxed feeling) was first described by the late Dr Herbert Benson, cardiologist, neuropsychologist, and creator of the Mind-Body Medicine programme at Harvard Medical School, as part of his seminal work in breathing techniques based around breathing in and out slowly. The response:

- Improves blood pressure control
- Breaks the train of everyday thoughts
- Helps you focus

- Helps you become self-aware
- Gives you more energy to succeed each day
- Reduces heart rate, blood pressure and increases parasympathetic tone

Mind-body medicine reduces heart disease, blood pressure, insomnia, arthritis, surgery recovery and low back pain. The GRACE and PEACE Massachusetts General Hospital studies showed that optimism reduces symptoms of angina and improves post-heart event recovery for patients. Gratitude increases exercise compliance. Gratitude interventions included:

- Practicing random acts of kindness and saying 'thank you'
- Remembering past success
- Writing a gratitude letter
- Reflecting
- Living by your personal strengths
- Undertaking enjoyable and meaningful activities

Do GRATITUDE Journal

> After I go to bed at night, I will take out my journal and write down three things for which I am grateful. Then I will smile and recall events. I will put journal away and go to sleep.
>
> The next morning, I will take out journal again and reflaection on what I wrote last night and recall one event that I am grateful for now and I will smile as I set up my new day.
>
> Do this for 30 days and see how you feel at end of 1 month.

Happiness is a better predictor of health risk than cholesterol levels. It is associated with longevity and quality of life in Blue Zone populations, especially in Denmark, Costa Rica and Singapore.

Happiness is:

- Living a life of purpose
- Altruism
- Gratitude
- Trust
- Economic growth
- Friendship
- Social connection
- Healthy diet
- Exercise
- Sleep
- Time out
- Spiritual health
- Energy and positive emotion
- Joy and pleasure – Whole Heart Health and a well-balanced life in its simplest form

How can I get into the habit of being more positive-minded and energetic? Pick actions such as those listed below to build on each day.

- Do an Acts of Loving Kindness meditation – check out videos on this on YouTube.
- Find purpose and do something you love doing every day.
- Say 'thank you' to everyone you meet.
- Practice gratitude: write thank-you notes and keep a gratitude journal.
- Leave the past in the past.
- Spend time outside absorbed in nature, get a pet or go for a walk.
- Have a laugh every day.
- Show love and appreciation.
- Concentrate on one task at a time.

- Learn to say 'no'.
- Avoid being triggered by stressful situations like sitting in traffic. Plan ahead by having a distraction podcast to listen to or practice mindful breathing or the relaxation response.
- Spend time around positive people and look at the positive in everything.
- Change your focus from negative to positive.
- Perform random acts of kindness, be generous to others, or do something new – try out new hobbies, e.g. painting.
- Take a day off, go for a massage and relax. I do this each month.
- Reach out to family and friends every day and spend time with them.
- Be part of a community – work, family, sports, hobbies and where you live.
- Celebrate all your small wins each time, every single day.
- Turn off the phone and take out the ear plugs.

These actions boost your brain's happy chemicals like dopamine, oxytocin and serotonin, which drive happiness and better health. They create inner calmness, lower stress, and better focus to help move you to achieving your goals. Pick *one* or *two* and start feeling more energetic now

Exercises for Self-Compassion, Gratitude and Positive Affirmations

Keep – a few minutes aside each day to pause and reflect
Prioritize – self-care, time out with self and loved ones
Pay – attention to present moment, enjoy the present moment
Practise – positive affirmations each day – I love myself, I am healthy and full of energy, I am a valuable team member, I contribute positively to my team every day
Have – daily team huddles where you check on each other's wellbeing and support each other
Debrief – after every incident at work to focus on wellbeing and supporting each other

LIMITING BELIEFS CAUSE HEART DISEASE

Limiting beliefs are beliefs that get into our head to sabotage our best efforts at making positive behaviour changes. We half-heartedly act and give up, citing excuses. This creates more negative beliefs and a vicious circle continues. This holds you back and stops your healthy behaviour change.

Ninety per cent of human thoughts, reactions, beliefs and behaviours are driven by the subconscious part of the brain. This can push you towards success as easily as holding you back. You choose.

Being calm and self-aware brings clarity and energy, and helps you to better understand how you think and believe, realising that some beliefs are deep down and were created unconsciously during childhood.

The solution to getting what you want lies in the story/narrative that you tell yourself. Ask yourself: 'Why am I holding back and what limiting belief is driving that?'

Reframing that story into a more positive, open narrative will boost your energy and help you to achieve the outcomes you want. But you must be fully committed and let your new dreams replace all your fears and limiting beliefs.

Health-related limiting beliefs may include:

- 'I do not have time' – 26 per cent of people think they do not have enough time to change their lifestyle.
- 'It is too expensive' – 17 per cent think this but fail to calculate the real financial cost of ill health.
- 'I am not able' – 27 per cent of people believe that they do not have the willpower, yet this is learned behaviour.
- 'I do not understand' – according to a US study, 52 per cent of Americans believe that it is easier to do taxes than to figure out how to eat healthily.

Health and life-limiting beliefs are entirely fear-based and there is a need to help people to shift to a healthier focused growth and abundance mindset. Each time fear comes up, be aware and change the narrative to the opposite positive thought. Get into this habit throughout each day.

- Awareness and self-discovery include identifying your limiting beliefs and allows you to heal.
- Rehearsing positive events and resources for 10–20 seconds throughout each day rewires the brain for happiness and resilience. It changes the mindset for heart health.
- Practicing daily gratitude mini-breaks helps to calm your brain and allows you to focus.
- Changing mindset takes time, so you cannot expect that doing these behaviours for two days here and there will make any difference to how you feel. In truth it takes at least 30 days for your brain to rewire from fear to optimism.

SIMPLE STEPS FOR ELIMINATING YOUR LIMITING BELIEFS: WELCOME, ACKNOWLEDGE AND RELEASE THEM

- Practice Box and Abdominal Breathing to ground you and focus, realising that what you believe is not true/real (this is known as Conscious Breathing). Breathe in for four seconds, hold for four seconds, breath out for four seconds, wait four seconds and start again. Increasing the out-breath duration will relax you more.
- Be more self-aware through your thinking and choosing. This can empower great health and happiness.
- Change 'I have to' to 'I get to'. Gratitude gives different energy. 'I get to exercise' vs 'I must exercise'. See how this makes you feel.

- Be up for a challenge, new opportunities and novel ways to tackle challenges and have self-belief.
- Do not get discouraged by failures: 'if you change the way you look at things, the things you look at change'. 'No' means 'next'. See failures as opportunities, be positive – you get to try again. Always tell yourself and believe that *you will* because you *can*.
- Do not play the victim game and blame others. Instead, tell yourself that things happen for a reason. See the positive, always.
- Do not wait for things to get better to be happy. Life will always be complicated. Learn to be happy now, otherwise you will run out of time. We want more, it is human. Acknowledge all the good you have and focus on being happy and living in the moment.
- Start small and grow. Keep calm and focus. Be compassionate and caring. Think balance, endurance, vision and courage.
- Cultivate self-compassion – this helps to combat perfectionism and self-criticism, be kind to yourself; change will not happen overnight, so be patient.
- Engage your beginner's mind – as if you know nothing, start anew, with a fresh perspective, uncover new opportunities. 'It is up to me.'
- Stop caring about what everyone else thinks.
- Dream big and ignore naysayers.
- Do not live in your own head – do not wish life away. Engage with the present.
- Be productive rather than busy
- Be creative, adaptable and unattached to the outcome.
- Search for unseen benefits – good things. Hope and take deep breaths. There is always silver to be found.
- Be with the right people – people who make you come alive. Stick with them and lose toxic people. If your three closest friends are overweight, then you have a 75% chance of becoming the same.

- Accept less than perfection – be grateful and happy with every chance you get, make peace with the idea that it is okay for things to be less than perfect. Accept a simplified life.
- Master your thoughts – change the voice in your head – put a name on your saboteur voice and say 'hello' and 'good-bye' as he/she appears. Instead of listening to 'I am worthless, useless, a failure,' change the voice.
- Empower yourself: 'Great job, well done.' See your problems as ways to grow!
- Take a compliment, be open and grateful.
- Use mantras and affirmations to help your awareness and to reduce stress. They should be positive and repeat every day four or five times. 'I am full of vitality and energy.' Listen to positive affirming music, videos and meditations. Keep these short and simple.
- Practice visualisations/stories (your own or source online) of positivity to take away fear and then use other tools with visualisations to remove all fears and limiting beliefs.
- Be compassionate, loving, mindful and do your best to avoid self-criticism. Let go of the past: 'my past does not dictate my future'.

There are many mind-based approaches to remove limiting beliefs and improve your physical health. They help you to have a more positive outlook on life and adopt healthier lifestyle habits by choice.

What are your limiting beliefs? Take a close look at the list and see what beliefs get in your way. Are these real for you and how do they affect your life choices? What steps can you take to change these beliefs? What goal would you like to achieve and what is stopping you? How can you get into the habit of letting these beliefs go? What action steps can you take now?

Start with one or two steps and grow. Pick one or two steps that resonate with you.

SECTION FOUR

Action Steps

9

The Science of Behaviour Change

Change is difficult. Most people (especially patients) find it easier to continue life as is, even when it comes at a personal cost to them. I have a patient who smokes 80 cigarettes every day, having saved €16,000 last year while he had stopped! The cost of his behaviour is not just financial, it affects everything in his life: its quality; its length; his risk of premature death, heart disease, lung cancer and permanent disability from breathing difficulties, stroke or even a leg amputation. Ironically, he does not smoke around his kids because he loves them and wants to be there for them. He says that 'he does not want to smoke and would like to stop and that is important to him, but not enough to stop his habit'. He has stopped smoking before and is unsure this time about whether he is able to stop again. His fears and limiting beliefs are consuming him.

Change only succeeds when it is easy, enjoyable and can be delivered in a simple, successful way. You must want to and have a burning desire to change. This might be the first time you have tried to make any meaningful change in your life and health.

The Transtheoretical Model of Change (TCM) is one well-published tool that has been applied to health behaviour programmes.

There are critics of the model that say it is flawed, the time periods are too arbitrary and vague, but the model is practical and easy to follow. There are five steps.

In my clinical practice, I combine TCM with the Health Behaviour Model and Fogg Behaviour Design Model. This gives structure to coaching behaviour change for the doctor and patient.

TRANSTHEORETICAL MODEL OF CHANGE

There are five steps in the transtheoretical model of change:

1. **Pre-contemplation** – Not ready. 'I can't.' Unmotivated to change.
2. **Contemplate** – Interested but not committed. Not confident. Ambivalent. 'I may.'
3. **Preparation** – 'I will.' Committed. Planning how to deal with obstacles.
4. **Action** – 'I am.' Taking action to cause change. Consistent. Positive feedback. Preventing relapse.
5. **Maintain** – 'I still am.' Successfully acting. Self-confident. Watch out for relapse.

Are you *ready* for change? By finding the right step, you will be able to identify actions you need to take.

How important is it for you to change now: 0–10?

How confident are you of success: 0–10?

0–3 = Not ready/Pre-contemplating

4–6 = Contemplating

7–8 = Preparation/Action

9–10 = Action/Maintain

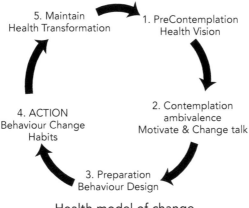

Health model of change

Step 1 – Precontemplation

This is the start point where most people are. 'I don't want to change or don't see a need to, as I don't have a problem.'

- In many cases, change is not thought out clearly or planned effectively.
- Health needs to be part of every day and people need to want to live that way.
- Change must be important enough so that the person is ready and able.
- Patients know there is a need to change but they do not know how to change and to sustain long-term, healthier ways of living.
- The focus is on daily behaviour not on outcomes.

Empowering people to transform their health behaviours is challenging. Motivation combined with emotion can bring about change talk and start conversations around change, followed by ongoing follow-up, but motivation alone does not last, primarily because it varies so much from person to person.

You can be motivated for a few days to stop smoking, but you find a cigarette and sneak off to have it, one puff and before you know it you are back to smoking every day. It is easier to lose your motivation than to sustain change. Eighty per cent of New Year's resolutions fail within 21 days.

Change needs to be easy to do and it needs to help patients succeed.

- All behaviour change plans must deal with any eventuality and have solutions in place to overcome reduced motivation.
- It is important to understand the environment that each person is in and how that is likely to affect behaviour success; being at home or being in work makes behaviour change different.
- Once the environment and prompting reminders are in place then change is likely to happen.
- It is not about perfection; it is about getting better.

As doctors, we give information to patients about health and some read it, but most do not, or they leave it in a drawer. We expect patients to understand complicated medical language. We need a simpler way to help patients to change their health behaviour.

People must understand (mind medicine) that their current lifestyle contributes to ill health and that change (action) is desirable. Ask the question:

- How interested are you in living? Enough to do something? If not, are you prepared to accept the consequences?
- What future do you want for yourself?
- How do you want to live/show up in life?
- Will you be able to walk and do your own shopping or to get down on the floor and play with your grandchildren?

I find this step empowers many patients to change lifelong poor habits like smoking.

How you want to live is what helps you to change your behaviour and your health. In clinic, I discuss heart attack health information to trigger contemplation and I ask patients to look at the risk to their health of not changing poor habits.

Self-awareness

Become self-aware of the inner story that you are telling yourself. What is stopping you from change? 'Why do I feel a resistance? What am I feeling? What thoughts/beliefs are holding me back?'
It is important to start from a position of strength. 'What am I good at? What is working?' Write down the stories you are telling yourself and see where changes might be possible. As you write these down, change will often happen.

Try addressing the following questions:

- Stories about your abilities and talents.
- Are stories helping, hurting, or giving you bigger options?
- What themes are coming up around your relationship with others?
- Are there old patterns that you would like to change?
- How would a slight change impact your life and work?
- Could you build a small daily habit that might help you make change happen?

Step 2 – Contemplation

In Step 2, you now know that you want to change and are open to it. But how?

- Pick a goal and behaviour, such as to lose weight by intermittent fasting from 7 p.m. to 7 a.m.
- Is your behaviour aligned with your goal?

- Is it easy to do and will it make you feel great doing it? This will build your confidence and momentum.
- Start with a small task such as eating one piece of fruit each day with breakfast.
- As you get used to this you can add more healthy eating behaviours each week.
- It is important to get the process working correctly before adding more small tasks.
- Starting with new behaviours is much easier than trying to replace old behaviours.
- If you want to change an existing behaviour like smoking, you must replace it with a new behaviour like drinking water/eating an apple.
- It helps to connect with your core values (see Appendices).
- Knowing your values helps you to sustain habits by doing what you love in the way you love to do it. This lowers stress levels.

Seeing positive health wins in front of your eyes every day is a brilliant motivator. Visualising your outcome (as if it is already happening) each day with positive emotion helps you to achieve sustained change. This focuses attention on your desired goal and daily repetition makes it happen. It combines the power of imagery of past, present and future, like travelling through time. Keep holding onto that feeling everyday of your goal already being achieved. That is the secret to long-lasting change.

Here is a simple example: find a comfortable quiet place where you will not be disturbed. Sit in a comfortable chair and close your eyes, breathe in gently for four seconds, hold for four, breath out for four and wait four seconds, then repeat three or four times.

Now, picture your future desired destination in the world, with a healthy version of you.

- What have you become?
- What are you doing?

- Where are you?
- How is your life different?
- How do you feel? (Take your time answering this one.)

Once these answers are clear to you, travel back to where you came from.

- Where did you stop on your way to the destination?
- What people did you meet and become friends with?
- Did you spend time together in clubs?
- Did you start new activities or hobbies?
- Did you take on a new career?
- Did you invent something?
- Spend as much time travelling back and forth and do this every day.

The final part of contemplation is getting a coach. In health this role is best overseen by your doctor. They may help you, guide you, motivate you and work with you.

Step 3 – Preparation

It is time for clarity. You want to change; you have small steps and are visualising your future self each day with joy and positive emotion. You have goals and you have picked a smaller goal to start with and one actionable step to take now.

It is important to have a Plan B to deal with any barriers/'what-ifs' that may arise, such as the WOOP (Wish, Outcome, Obstacle, Plan) Method. This helps you to overcome obstacles and achieve longer lasting change. Ideally you will not need to use Plan B as you are focused on having Plan A already happen!

- WOOP is based on Implementation Intention – a psychological strategy that forces people to confront how they will address obstacles that get in their way.
- Obstacles: 'What is the obstacle that is holding you back from change?'
- Plan: Create a plan. What can you do to overcome your obstacle? Find one small step. 'If there is an obstacle then I will take a small step/action/thought,' e.g. 'If I am hungry between meals then I will pause and breathe for 20 seconds and celebrate.'
- You can journal all potential obstacles and ways around them as you want and then practice the small steps multiple times each day until it feels right for you.
- Try to stay focused on the small steps and do not drift into big goals.
- Meditation and breathwork can help you to do that. Get this consistently right and progress will happen. This will give you positive feedback and drive change.
- Sometimes it is about tackling this one day at a time. Have fun with what you are doing as emotions convert behaviours into habits.

Motivational Interviewing

Many patients (and quite a few doctors) are not able to make all these instructions happen and coaching techniques such as motivational interviewing can help. Motivational interviewing is a collaborative, goal-orientated style of communication with particular attention to the language of change. It is designed to strengthen personal motivation for and commitment to a specific goal by eliciting and exploring the person's own reasons for change within an atmosphere of acceptance and compassion.

What is fluctuating is how to act in accordance with that insight (will power). Positive effects on will power are often achieved indirectly as clarity gained in good coaching contributes to strengthen self-confidence, better awareness of one's values and better overall wellbeing.

Behaviour Design

Re-engineering patient behaviour (making change easier) is a practical way to reduce the amount of will power that is necessary for implementing new habits.

Rather than depending on the fluctuating degree of will power that is available at any given moment to act on cognitive insight, patients are taught how to design new health behaviours, health routines and to build habits that are independent of will power – requiring a minimum of will power in the process. Work *smarter*, not harder; be consistent; make tasks easy and make sure you feel great and successful doing the behaviour. Make behaviour easy to do and you will feel success (so it motivates you). This will deliver change when the action is triggered so that you keep remembering to do it.

Step 4 – Action

- Visualise your goal as already achieved and what that looks and feels like. Keep at it until you have achieved your goal. Affirm and be grateful for being healthy now. Hold that vision in your mind, feel your success and it will manifest in your hands through the action and habits you create and follow. (Look at Novak Djokovic's interview after winning the French Open Tennis in 2023 and note how he visualised it since he was seven years old. Listen to how he visualises every shot of the match beforehand as well.) This is how you prime yourself for success. Focus on the goal and remove any distractions.

- Make the behaviour enjoyable, consistent and fun to do. Experiment and get creative to find what works best. Visualisation makes the desired behaviour easier to do.
- Make time every day to do your new behaviours.
- Celebrating each small step primes our brains to repeat behaviours due to positive feedback.
- Pick the celebration that you enjoy most, like a smile, a dance, a thumbs up or a fist pump as examples (something that lifts your energy level). Pick one of these and make it yours.
- Practicing gratitude in everything you do, drives your subconscious mind.

Changing some of these factors will make it easier for you to succeed.. If you want to start tennis as a new exercise, then you will need to buy tennis shoes, tennis balls and a racket to play with. Ask yourself: 'Can I change my environment to make the behaviour easier?'

You must remember to do the behaviour. It is easy to forget or to get distracted. For example, you decide to start running. You get all the running clothes and go out for ten minutes on Saturday and Sunday. Then you work all week and next Saturday it is raining so you skip running and on Sunday you are tired so you miss it as well. By the following week, you have given up running altogether.

It might be easier to start smaller with one-minute runs each day to get into the routine of running. When the routine is in place then it is the time to stack more behaviours, such as running faster or further.

Do not beat up yourself for having a difficult day. Accept that this happens and start afresh the next day. Do not let the inner critic drive negative emotions such as fear. These thoughts include:

- All-or-nothing thinking – yes or no
- Overgeneralising – never-ending failure
- Negative mental filter – dwelling on negatives

- Jumping to conclusions – predicting bad outcomes or assuming everyone hates you without any objective evidence (think and see what you want before taking action)

How you deal with your thoughts and beliefs are critical to sustaining change. Being self-aware of your inner consciousness and thought patterns helps you to learn how to deal with them in a positive way. You can let go and move forward with ease. This is your change in thinking (nothing will stop you now!) which often happens by just doing the small steps and experiencing the joy and emotion that brings, thus shifting your mood instantly.

A straightforward way to overcome any resistance to exercising is to start identifying tasks that you do every day, such as waking up or getting out of bed. This can be a reminder for you to do healthy behaviour. This is called a trigger, or a prompt. It must be specific and dependable because without a prompt, a behaviour cannot happen. You can use an existing activity like getting out of bed or design a context prompt like after your alarm clock goes off, or Alexa reminds you, or try a mental prompt (you try to remember to do it).

It is important that the trigger is clear to the person doing the behaviour:

- Does the prompt work? Is it the best way to prompt the person to do the new behaviour?
- You can also choose to be healthy all day and practice related behaviours at any opportunity you have. Instead of sitting at your desk all day, stand up every 10 minutes.
- Your beginner's mindset impacts success. Hold the dream in your mind all day: see it, feel it, take steps forward and it will manifest.
- Feeling good, growth, love, optimism and gratitude get the job done.

- Putting positive emotions into or celebrating every moment that you do these behaviours helps them to become a habit. Behaviours that are easy to do and are enjoyable become habitual.
- Behaviour changes can be made as one-off actions, timed over weeks/months, or made as permanent choices to form habits.
- You must keep doing the same new behaviour every day (consistently) as a new routine and you might forget to do it unless you like doing it.
- It is easier to undo progress in as little as one week so we must keep at the new routine every day.

If struggling, then reflect on why.

- Your beliefs and values – are they aligned?
- What is stopping you from doing the behaviour thoughts?
- Are you trying too hard?
- Do you need to make the behaviour smaller or easier to do, like a two-minute run instead of ten minutes?
- Do you need to change it because it is not for you and then you must find something else to do to reach your goal?
- Have you got a prompt? Is it working?
- Do you like the behaviour you are trying to do?

Follow some ideas below to help you succeed:

- Is the behaviour easy to do? If not, why?
- How can you make the behaviour easier for you to do?
- Do you need to learn how or get someone to help or train you?
- Are you clear on what you want to achieve by doing this behaviour?
- Are you clear what you are to do, how, where, and when? If not, ask for help. You can ask your coach or doctor and build a

plan that answers all these questions and puts you on the right track to success.

In practice, most people do not have a clear plan in place, or they forget the trigger, or they are not emotionally invested in doing the behaviour. Stories, distractions, resistance and limiting beliefs creep in. Several people do not have any trigger, so they are not interested in making any change to health behaviour. Their solution might be triggering health concerns.

Tips for making behaviour change easier:

- Dream up big goals, visualise achieving them now, affirm this and be grateful. Do the behaviours to build new healthy habits.
- Have a written starting plan that anticipates problems and has ways for you to deal with resistance.
- I find that giving out instructions/prescriptions journal to patients is a great starting point for triggering behaviour change and starting a new routine.
- Some people respond better to written or short video prompts.
- Messaging apps may also work.

Once patients are comfortable with the new health routine, they can add or stack more behaviours or try new prescriptions that involve other behaviours or lifestyle pillars.

My most successful coaching approach is to:

- Trigger patients with a kickstart plan based around their health goal
- Coach weekly
- Communicate weekly or less based on the client
- I like to introduce the kickstart plan when patients are in front of me at a clinic and are focused on health.
- As you try to change you need to take time every day to reflect on and review progress. The purpose is to help increase your

awareness of why you are doing this, to slow down and to see if you need to make changes.

- Some like to write a list in their journal of 3–5 tasks to be done on the next day.
- It is essential that you switch off at night, turn off devices, screens, relax, sleep and recharge for the following day. Be grateful for your successes each day and for what is to come tomorrow.
- It is equally important that you are not overeating, or drinking too much alcohol and/or coffee that will disrupt your sleep recovery as well as your health.
- Getting into the right frame of mind every day is also critical.

Tony Robbins uses a priming routine of cold bath/shower, meditation, breathing exercises and a positive visualisation exercise to get him into his peak physiological state to face each day. You need this awakening to focus your mind and to kick start each day. I get into a warm shower and then switch the dial to cold for a minute or two. I find that is my kickstart to face the day ahead with energy and excitement. Then I continue in a way that I want, focusing on the goal I want to achieve that day.

Step 5 – Maintain

Positive emotions turn behaviours into habits. These actions have created new healthy habits and you are feeling and looking great. You are transforming yourself and your health. Well done and keep at it.

There is still a risk of relapse: 15 per cent of people will go back to step one, but 85 per cent will eventually return to the action step. It is important to avoid anxiety, procrastination and stress that may derail progress.

- What is stressing you?
- What is going on around you?
- What is happening to make you more stressed? Write these down.
- Examine why they are stressful and how you can overcome this and plan for this by creating coping strategies.

There are multiple actions that you can take (see the last chapter). Look at your use of time and what you could do instead. Learn to say no. Get support from friends, colleagues and loved ones.

- Build your motivation and confidence through small steps.
- Reconnect with your values (see Appendices).
- Visualise your 'why', your goals and having achieved them.
- Tap into your positive emotions: what makes you feel good and full of energy.
- Learn and iterate: refine your goal, continue to challenge yourself and your progress. These will build confidence. Celebrate this.
- Get support from friends and others who are on the same journey.
- Meet up, support each other emotionally, give accountability and brainstorm new ways forward.

Helping Patients to Get into Healthy Habits

10

Heart Health Behaviour Design

As doctors we prescribe medications to manage cholesterol, blood pressure, diabetes, to keep stents open, to stabilise plaque in arteries, to control irregular heartbeats and to treat heart failure. We give instructions about when to take medications, how many times per day, for how long and we highlight potential side effects with use. We assume patients will take the medications.

In other cases, we prescribe healthy activities like FITT (Frequency, Intensity, Time and Type of activity) prescriptions to empower patients to exercise but we do not include how to keep doing the behaviour. This might be to walk for five days per week at low intensity for 30 minutes, for example. In the context of small steps, we often ask patients to do too much.

- Healthy Habits prescriptions are a useful tool that remind patients to start small changes in health behaviours. This could be walking for one minute each day after parking the car.
- I usually prescribe one small behaviour for patients to do each day, e.g. gratitude journaling three times per day.

111

- They can increase the duration or intensity as they go but I encourage a gradual pace.
- Then I follow up at the next clinic / coaching visit.
- Patients can contact me for support as needed or I will call them to see how they are doing if I do not hear from them.

Male patients will frequently try too hard when starting to exercise, forcing them to quit or causing injury. This will trigger poor eating habits, disrupted sleep and inevitable stress returning because they are annoyed or in pain from their injury.

Patients are more compliant when they have clear instructions. Improved results are possible with support from the patient's pharmacy or their doctor if side effects or questions arise. Tracking blood results for effect or measuring weight, blood pressure and heart rate for feedback, as well as seeing their doctor for ongoing follow-up, also improve results.

CHECKING YOUR BLOOD PRESSURE

I use the Habits Prescription approach with patients to check their blood pressure at home:

'At each mealtime (your trigger to do the desired behaviour), I will sit down at the kitchen table and measure my blood pressure and write down the reading.'

They can then send a week of results directly to me or bring them to the clinic.

The only way that this can work is where each patient:

- Knows when to do the behaviour (after sitting at the breakfast table they put the BP cuff on)
- Knows the behaviour (to put BP cuff on) and
- Is emotionally involved (celebrates) – they feel success because they are doing the BP check and they can smile about that!

The patient will only remember what to do and what the readings are by keeping a written record. My Blood Pressure Habits prescription is designed this way.

In the example of blood pressure readings, I am looking at patterns to adjust a patient's medications and to understand their behaviours to better control the blood pressure. This helps patients to understand that we can add/stack more new health behaviours after they check their blood pressure in the morning, such as drinking a glass of water!

As you can see, the health habit prescription is triggering patients to change behaviour and start a new routine; it is helping people design behaviours to make health and self-care easier to do all the time as well as reminding patients to do these behaviours and build a new routine.

The blood pressure habit could be substituted with checking your blood sugar before each meal every day, or whatever is suitable in your situation.

A prescription is a straightforward way to prompt you to do the behaviour and it gives instructions on what behaviour you are to do. You might need to make a smaller step to prompt yourself to read the prescription, such as after you get out of bed, or you can put a post-it on your bathroom mirror. You might need to leave the blood pressure machine on the kitchen table! The more frequently that you do the behaviour, the sooner it becomes habitual. Do not forget to celebrate that you are carrying out these great healthy steps and to visualise your new, healthy self each day. Habits are established by enjoying the behaviours.

II

Health Habit Kickstart Prescriptions

Getting into the habit of better lifestyle health can be prescribed based around the six pillars of better sleep, less stress, healthy eating, physical activity, social connection, and stopping addiction.

KICKSTART HEALTH HABIT PRESCRIPTION FOR HEALTHY EATING

Dr name and qualification   Date

Patient Name, address, date of birth

Rx

After sitting down for breakfast, lunch and dinner DRINK ONE Glass of water, then celebrate with a smile.

Do this each day for 21 days.

Keep record of progress / snags

Dr signature

Please contact doctor's office if you are struggling to do this on 01-0000

HAPPY MIND PRESCRIPTION

(Instructions for Use: Do this behaviour every morning. Write it down, repeat for 30 days and feel free to add more behaviours that help you feel amazing each morning. Keep a journal to recall, even read it back to yourself each night. Remember to start small and take your time. One day and one habit at a time and get it right. Your purpose is being healthy every day. Celebrate each behaviour as you complete it.)

- After I get out of bed I will say 'It's going to be an amazing day,' and smile.
- After I get into the shower, I will turn on the cold tap and smile.
- After I brush your teeth, I will look at my great self in the mirror, smile and celebrate.

PRESCRIPTION FOR BETTER SLEEP

- After I come home from work, I will turn the phone on airplane mode and celebrate.
- After I finish dinner, I will go out for a gentle five-minute walk and celebrate.
- After I lie on my pillow, I will do breathing exercises/meditate and celebrate.

PRESCRIPTION FOR HEALTHIER EATING

- After I sit down for breakfast I will pause, take a breath and celebrate.
- After I sit down for meals, I will drink a large glass of water and celebrate.
- After I feel 80 per cent full of food, I will put my knife and fork down and celebrate.

Do as instructed, keep a record daily, weigh yourself weekly, feel free to add more healthy eating habits such as eating fruit and vegetables, using a smaller plate/taking smaller portion sizes, replacing sugary and salty foods with healthier options and remember to take your time and small steps.

PRESCRIPTION FOR BEING MORE PHYSICALLY ACTIVE (INCLUDING STARTING PHYSICAL ACTIVITY)

- After I park my car, I will put on my runners/walking shoes, take a five-minute walk and celebrate (do this at work and when home in the evening).
- After I get out of bed, I will do two push-ups and celebrate.
- After I get up from using the toilet, I will do two squats and celebrate.

Feel free to increase numbers as you succeed but do not jump from 2 to 100 habits, gradually increase. Keep a daily record and track your heart rate/steps if you wish. If walking, start very slowly, take small steps and short distances and build up slowly each day/week.

PRESCRIPTION FOR LOWERING STRESS

- After I lie down on my pillow, I will write down five things that I am grateful for in my journal and smile before I go to sleep.
- After I meet people, I will say 'thank you' and smile.
- After a negative thought comes to mind, I will have a laugh and celebrate.
- After I wake up, I will visualise and affirm a stress-free day ahead and celebrate.

Again, do these every day, keep a record in your diary, monitor how you feel each day (happier/not), feel free to add more stress-lowering behaviours as you go and refer to earlier chapters for behaviours that lower your stress levels or make you feel happy.

KICKSTART IN ACTION – DOING YOUR PRESCRIBED BEHAVIOURS EVERY DAY

These healthy habits can be prescribed for any length of time and then followed up with the doctor for review. Keeping a record of doing daily habits on a 30-day calendar helps to reinforce behaviour change. Alternatively, use an Excel spreadsheet.

- Sharing what you are doing, and why, with your family, spouse, friends and getting them involved increases your likelihood of long-term behaviour change success.
- If you forget to do the behaviour, then your day one starts again the next day.
- Keeping a league table among friends or family can bring a gaming element to your behaviour challenge and keep people active and involved.
- The objective is getting started and growing every day to achieve sustained behaviour change. Make a personal commitment to do the new behaviour tomorrow.
- The how-to-use instructions are the same for all habit prescriptions.
- They are reviewed at monthly intervals and we troubleshoot any problems.

I ask that patients who are struggling get in touch with my office.

Each person will differ in terms of doing new behaviours, changing existing behaviours and stopping certain behaviours. If I have no contact from these patients every few days, I will contact the patient directly to see what is going on.

The overall objective for each patient is to:

- Learn how to do the new behaviour.
- Know what to do.
- Start doing the behaviour in small incremental steps and to celebrate immediately as you take each small step. Yippee!
- Build a routine with time.
- Practice until perfect, supported by coaching with weekly feedback and journaling.
- Stack more healthy behaviours as you establish new habits.
- Achieve the SMART goal that you created. Focus on one goal at a time.
- You must align all new healthier behaviours with your values and desired health outcomes to improve heart health such as reversing diabetes, weight issues, cholesterol, lowering blood pressure.
- Over time, patients master their behaviour routine and it becomes a habit through positive associated emotions.
- All of this only happens with patience and practice.
- Getting feedback and having dedicated support (e.g. greater accountability partners from family, friends or work colleagues) helps to sustain the behaviour change.
- Coaching over the long term is essential.
- Visualise, positively affirm success and be grateful for achieving your dream goal each day.

The clinical evidence for effective long-term behaviour change interventions has been reported by academic and technology groups. Ancora Health in Holland showed that meaningful lifestyle behaviour change, based on the Fogg Model, can be sustained at twelve months. They measure lifestyle changes like healthy eating, supported by digital in-person and group coaching, patient monitoring and a mobile app for journaling and providing health information.

The COACH Australia study in heart disease patients showed that lifestyle behaviour change can be achieved (by adopting similar tools) for five years.

Certain behaviour change approaches are associated with longer-lasting change in clinical populations. These include:

- *Positive* motivation – instead of self-criticism. Empowering patients matters
- Having a clear *plan* of action and ways to overcome any barriers
- Using *goal* setting and aligning with patient core *values* and a clear purpose
- Approaches that are coach-led and supported
- Repeated learning for the patient with feedback
- Accountability – from a spouse, mentor or role model
- Patient information is provided
- Patient, environment/context and the behaviour are clearly understood and applied
- Self-efficacy is driven by joy/emotion gained from new behaviours/habits plus results achieved (positive feedback)

12

Steps to Achieving Your Individual Health Goals

Goal: 'I will run a 10 km charity race in 50 minutes on 1 July 2024'

- What is your current level of activity?
- What do you like doing?
- What are you able to do? What is stopping you from exercising?
- What are you hoping to achieve?
- How important is that to you? Rank 0–10 (low to high importance).
- How confident are you about achieving your goal (0–10)?
- What will help you to achieve your goal? What is stopping you from that? Find the tools you need.
- What exercise behaviours are easy for you to do and what will make you feel success (becoming healthier, trying to line up a 5 km run, losing weight) in doing this? Walk, run, swim, tennis, hill-walking. What are you doing at the moment in terms of exercise?

- How will you remember to do some exercise every day?
- How can you make it fun and easy to do at every step?
- Visualise yourself running 2 km and what that feels like. Where are you? What gear are you wearing? Are you measuring heart rate and distance? See yourself crossing the finish line, feeling amazing and healthier. Affirm that you are so happy and grateful for doing this. Use these tools to programme your mind that you are healthy and then it can help you act that way.

Start with a small goal – walk ten minutes each night after dinner. Goal-setting will help you to reach your dreams of being healthy and disease-free. I start each day with a plan as to how I am going to be healthy that day, such as walking for ten minutes each day.

SMARTER goal-setting is your best approach.

- **S**pecific: such as I will walk for ten minutes each day after I get dressed in the morning.
- **M**easurable: how successful are you? Get a calendar and tick off progress each day, marking 'Yes' or 'No'.
- **A**ttainable: take small steps that are simple and easy to do. This will make you feel successful in doing them. Start small, move slowly and grow.
- **R**ealistic: only set goals that you know you will be able to achieve. Walk before running. Slow progress vs fast failure.
- **T**ime-orientated: pick a time frame to complete your goal. Have a short end in sight, such as in one week. You might like to enter a short race as motivation or time your exercise pace and track your progress like walking a further distance within your ten minutes than at the start. This will help to make it habitual.
- Go **E**asy on yourself and start small so that you **R**epeat the behaviours each day.

Week one aim: 'I will walk for ten minutes each evening after I park my car outside home.'

- If you prefer, you can change the time at which to go (make it as easy and as much fun as you can): you might choose after getting out of bed or at any other trigger time.
- Then put on your walking shoes, clothes and go for a walk for ten minutes.
- You might want to check what the weather is like so you can dress appropriately.
- After the ten minutes, stop, celebrate that you did it and go home. Or do an extra two minutes.
- If you are new to the activity, then start with increases of one- or two-minutes duration and build up more slowly.
- Be aware of your usual daily routine so you can find enough time to do the walking.
- Block time out in your calendar.
- Ensure you have the right shoes.
- Ensure you have a road map of where you are going.
- Are you able to walk?
- Do you want to do the walk?
- Make sure that nothing else is going to get in the way.
- Always use the habits prescription to kickstart your new behaviour: 'After I get out of bed in morning, I will put on my walking gear and go for a ten-minute walk and celebrate'.
- Start there, get the routine right and then you can increase the walking duration as your days/weeks progress.
- Alternatively, you could do ten sets of one-minute exercises each day, such as using the stairs, walking to the bus stop, doing squats or sit-ups. This way gives variety and fun as well as encouraging healthy steps all day.
- Write down what you achieved and celebrate that action too.
- Do not forget to relax.

- Be grateful for your walk and visualise what being healthy and heart-disease-free feels like to you now. Do that on every walk.
- Keep well hydrated.
- After your walk, head home for a shower and take your tablets or do another health-minded behaviour that aligns with your goals/vision, such as checking your blood pressure or eating a healthy bowl of porridge.
- Celebrate every action so that these new health behaviours become habits and write them down every single day so you can see your progress and reinforce your daily effort.
- For walking you could arrange to get someone to go with you/collect you each morning. This is good for friendship, socialisation and keeping you accountable. You and your friend could plan new activities and try those as well. You might reach out to community, join a local walking group, football club or men's shed. Get others involved.
- Remember that you know what you can do, so pace yourself. Do not overdo it as you will not enjoy that, and it will block your interest in going for your next walk/run.
- Your new heart condition may affect this so take your time. Ask your doctor for advice if you need guidance. Follow the Habit Prescription as your doctor has instructed and stick with the plan.
- Bear in mind that it may take a month or two to make exercise a new habit, but keep doing it no matter what, even if it is just stepping outside in shoes for two minutes, especially on a day when you are lacking in motivation.
- Add extra goals as you go – stretching, toning or balance routines, yoga, or meditation. If you do not know, ask someone, or look for short easy-to-do actions on YouTube.
- Journal your progress every day. Use a 30-day calendar to keep a record by ticking or marking an 'X' on each day that you complete the task. How do you feel?

- Remember that being inactive increases your risk of a heart attack by over 11 per cent.
- You could take the opportunity to add more heart healthy behaviours into your routine, like checking your weight each morning after your shower. (This could be discussed with the doctor to help you stack healthy-eating behaviours as one of the next goals, in addition to your exercise rituals. Getting this right will help with any blood pressure, cholesterol, diabetes problems and transform your heart health.) Whatever you decide to do, always take things slowly and take small steps first.
- You can monitor your progress with measures of activity intensity, heart rate, the talk test, trackers or watches. My advice, however, is to get started first and then grow, instead of spending money joining a gym or buying gadgets when what you most need is comfortable shoes and putting one foot in front of the other first.
- It may help to replace inactivity with doing something physically active – write down all the ways that you could reduce inactivity and replace those behaviours with more active behaviours (turning the TV off, limiting your time on the computer). You could reduce time spent doing nothing or do some other healthy behaviour instead. Do this every day until you see changes happening in your life.
- Add variety to your physical activity as you get more active. Keep it interesting and find what you like and want to repeat. Maybe cycle to work instead of driving, take a flight of stairs at work instead of using the lift, bring lunch to work instead of going to the cafeteria. Be creative as you find new health behaviours to add in and have fun doing this.
- Celebrate your new behaviours and reward your goals with something healthy like buying a new pair of walking shoes or Fitbit/smart watch, joining an exercise class or visiting the gym. In France you can donate to a charity app as you become healthier. Get a friend to join you for fun and support.

- Cardiac rehab may introduce you to new heart friends who could help you plan for success. You can achieve greatness by sticking with it and giving as much at the end as in the beginning. If you are struggling, get help immediately from a nurse/physiotherapist/doctor or gym trainer. The longer you procrastinate the more damage you are doing to your heart.
- Bring your records and journal with you when you return to see the doctor/cardiologist to assess your progress and goal achievement and to see how your health is improving. This will help the doctor to build on your existing plan and keep your goals aligned with improving your heart health.

You can model the approach of the Physical Activity Plan for other lifestyle pillars such as improving your sleep, lowering stress or eating healthier.

HEALTHY EATING PLAN

Goal: 'To lose two stone in weight in the next 90 days by ...'

Write this goal down and make it SMART. Visualise a two-stone-lighter body on the date that is in 90 days' time. Wow! How do you look and feel? Where are you? What are you wearing? How do your clothes feel on you? See yourself in front of a mirror, jumping for joy. 'I did it, I released two stone in weight from my body.' Celebrate your success with affirmations of how happy and grateful you are. Celebrate your progress towards being healthier. Do this every day as often as you like. Programme your brain to feel healthy and that will make habits easier to form and do.

Healthy Eating Plan:
- Take a photograph of your current self.
- Visualise what being healthy will feel like for you when you are two stone lighter.
- Set a goal of releasing two pounds in weight per week for twelve weeks by eating smaller food portions and engaging in other healthy eating behaviours.
- Start by eating smaller portions of food daily.
- Choose eating behaviours that are easy to do and will help you lose weight:
  » Drink water with meals
  » Mindful eating at each meal – go slowly
  » Fast from 7.00 p.m. to 7.00 a.m. or later the next day (intermittent fasting)
  » Pick a more balanced healthy plate mix of protein, carbohydrate and fats
  » Drink less alcohol
  » Reduce sugar intake
- See a dietician
- Weigh your food

- Prepare lunch the night before for the next day, or make batches of foods for the next week
- Sign up to a healthy meal delivery service
- Eat five vegetables and two fruit each day
- Fill your fridge with healthy food only
- Count calories daily, and keep intake to the recommended amount for your age and body size
- Listen to motivating music
- Do exercise
- Eat with family and turn phones off
- Start with one or two behaviours first, get the routine right and then add another behaviour
- You can trigger the healthy eating behaviours at mealtimes, like 'After I sit down to the breakfast table, I will drink a glass of water.' You may need another habit to leave the glass on the table – 'After I walk into the kitchen, I will set the table for my breakfast with …', thus making it easy and rewarding (being healthy) to do these behaviours. Celebrate each behaviour and make them habits
- Monitor food intake each day; you will feel clothes getting bigger on you
- Weigh yourself once per week
- Get friends and family to collaborate with you
- Keep a daily journal and review it each evening: how did today go and what steps are you going to take tomorrow?
- Add walking or gratitude journaling to each day
- If you are struggling, remember to keep trying, one difficult day is allowed but never two
- Be positive every day (visualise, affirm, engage in positive self-talk and reframe)
- Be confident and you will get there
- Meet up with your friends, share your experiences and support each other
- Make a goal to be healthy by doing these behaviours each day

BETTER NIGHT'S SLEEP PLAN

Goal: 'To be refreshed in the morning by sleeping for seven hours each night for the next 30 days'

Visualise waking up every day healthy, rested, fully recovered, energetic and enthusiastic. You feel amazing. Be happy and grateful and remind yourself of this all day. Visualise the new behaviours that are helping you feel this way such as a new pillow!

Better Sleep Plan:
- Set a goal of sleeping for at least seven hours every night for 30 days by going to bed at a fixed time
- Eat earlier
- Relax for one hour before bed
- Meditate
- Create a time cut-off for turning off the mobile phone, studying, working and watching exciting TV shows
- Stay awake during the day
- Set the bedroom temperature
- Ensure the bedroom is quiet and comfortable
- Do you need a special pillow/mask/earplugs or a blue light cover?
- Reduce noise level
- Stop coffee intake after 2.00 p.m.
- Limit chocolate intake
- Limit alcohol intake
- Eat your main meal at lunchtime
- Beware when taking paracetamol, not to take one with added caffeine
- Spend time outside during the day
- Keep a regular sleep schedule throughout the whole week
- Avoid exercise in the late evening, especially after a busy workday
- Stop smoking and avoid drinking too much fluids late at night

- Start with one behaviour only and establish your new healthy sleep routine
- Prompt the bedtime sleep routines with examples, such as deciding that after eating dinner I will turn my phone to airplane mode
- Decide that: 'After dinner I will start a wind-down behaviour, take a shower, have my camomile tea and lie down in bed.' You could set an alarm to prompt you. You could then do a gratitude habit in bed that helps celebrate the momentous day and sets you up for less stress in the days ahead as well
- Monitor sleep duration each night
- You could use a wearable device such as Firstbeat
- Keep a journal of your progress
- You will want to adjust behaviours that help you sleep better
- Ask friends and family to collaborate with you
- Add walking or gratitude journaling to each day
- If you are struggling to find a better sleep routine, remember to keep trying. One difficult day is allowed but never two. Be positive every day (practice visualising what it feels like when you are sleeping perfectly and affirm, engage in positive self-talk and reframe). Be confident and you will get there
- Meet up with your friends, share your experience and support each other

LOWER STRESS LEVELS PLAN

Goal: 'To be happy and energetic every day for 21 days'

Or you could set a goal of doing a gratitude journal each night for 30 days and measure your level of happiness on day 1 and day 30.

Look at your sleep plan and imagine a visualisation for this pillar ... sit back and close your eyes. What does being happy and grateful for life, health and family look and feel like for you? Feel the emotion and what that does to you and for your health. Imagine that you are stress-free and feeling amazing. Visualise, affirm this. Keep a journal, write in it, and reflect on how great you feel, and read it back.

Stress Reduction Plan:

There are multiple behaviours to pick from, that increase your positivity, give you energy, and help you to see the plus in everything:

- Breathe: do box breathing (breathe in for four seconds, hold for four, breath out for four and rest for four), or belly breathing (as you breathe in, push your tummy out and as you breathe out bring your tummy back in; put your hand on your tummy to feel the air moving in, then moving out and in again). Do this after you wake up each day for one month.
- Meditate for two minutes after the shower each morning for one month
- Look after other lifestyle pillars
- Leave the past behind
- Savour good things
- Say thank you
- Be grateful
- Practice gratitude
- Do random acts of kindness

- Get a pet
- Talk with family and friends
- Go for a walk every day
- Have a laugh
- Show love and appreciation
- Focus on one task at a time
- Slow down – find your mind's imaginary quiet place and spend some time there
- Say 'no'
- Practice time management
- Stand up every 15 minutes
- Let go and declutter your mind of thoughts
- Reward yourself
- Be kind to others
- Do something new
- Write out all the remarkable things in life
- Use your inner strengths
- Listen to motivating music
- Do a happy habits hour each morning
- Go for a massage
- Take a day off
- Celebrate every small win each day
- Practice, practice, practice
- Prioritise self-care first
- Prompting stress reduction can be: 'After I wake up in the morning I will say "it's going to be an impressive day" and smile.' 'After I lie down in bed at night, I will write three things in my journal that I am grateful for.'
- You could make a stress scale of 0–10 and score your happiness and energy levels each day, say in the morning and evening. You can start with two to three behaviours and see how you get on with those. Do they make you feel more or less happy? Should you change these behaviours?
- Keep at it for 30 days and see how you feel.

- Practising gratitude is the best habit for lowering stress.
- Get other people involved such as workmates, family, friends and see how everyone can benefit. Keep a journal and if you are struggling make behaviour smaller or just stick to one behaviour.

Review your progress each day and revise it for the next day as needed. Commit to doing the new behaviour again tomorrow. Being healthy is a choice, a way of living, to prevent heart disease and to treat/reverse chronic diseases and risk factors. Choosing this will guide you to a longer and happier life.

SECTION SIX

Mastering Your Heart Health

13

Simple Steps for Being Healthy Every Day

1. Imagine what being healthy every day means for you. Close your eyes, ground your breath with five minutes of box breathing and centre yourself. Think: what does being healthy mean to you? What would you really like to achieve? What is your burning desire? What is your big health goal? What pillar of lifestyle do you want to work on? Eating, exercise, stress, sleep, smoking, drinking, connecting with family and friends?

2. Practice positive affirmations daily: 'I am so happy and grateful now that I am healthy'; 'I am living in a healthy body'; 'I weigh X pounds'; 'I am eating fresh, healthy food'; 'I am drinking two litres of water every day'; 'I go to bed early'; 'I am sleeping peacefully'; 'I am free of stress and I am full of energy'; 'I am healthy.' Keep it simple. Pick two or three and repeat the affirmations every day for 30 days.

3. What behaviours are needed to achieve your healthy goal? Look at the lifestyle medicine habits. Where do you start?

Pick one behaviour that is easy to do and will make you feel healthier doing it. Perhaps choose going for a walk each night to become physically active or to help lose weight.

4. What steps do you need to take? Think of five steps to make the behaviour easy to do: shoes, music, pick route, clothing, time, get a walking friend or pet. Start with walking for a few minutes and then increase slowly each evening. Celebrate your walk immediately afterwards with a smile, high-five or whatever lifts your emotions. Well done, you did it!

5. Keep a record of how you did and felt. Hydrate. You might increase the distance of your next walk. Set that as a new goal. Choose a slight increase, such as half-a-mile.

6. Keep visualising and affirming your goal already achieved every day, and feel how that makes you feel to achieve your goal. Practice a gratitude habit each day and be kind to yourself. Celebrate every healthy behaviour as you complete them. Feel how that makes you feel and enjoy that. This emotional step is critical to your success

7. Build confidence and schedule an action each day. Be grateful and get into the habit of doing all of these steps every day and keeping a written record of it.

8. Persist, have faith, and keep doing it every day until it becomes an established habit. Do not give up. Come to realise that you are now healthy every day and that you live that way.

14

Troubleshooting Health Behaviour Design

Successful behaviour change depends on your emotional state activating your subconscious mind: what are your beliefs, your thoughts, your story/imagination, your feelings and what is your effective action plan for becoming healthy?

If change is not happening for you then something is not working. There will always be a clear explanation that you can address. Start looking at your thoughts instead of pushing harder on your actions. This will depress you and bring limiting beliefs to the surface.

You must be emotionally connected (feeling good) to behaviour change to make it habitual. You need the right attitude (thinking, positive feeling, believing, being grateful and doing the right habits) to make change happen. You have to feel amazing from your goal and vision of your ideal health. Then do the behaviours that are fun to do and you enjoy doing. In this way it is easy to build new health habits.

Celebrating each behaviour is part of that emotion. If you are unhappy, your story is likely to counteract your plans for change.

But if you respond to that unhappiness with high energy by being positive then the outcome will be different. One trick is to welcome the unhappiness with open arms, embrace it, and realise everything is going to be fine. At that point, true happiness is going to appear.

Sometimes people get started and then stop. Other times, they cannot start and cannot work out why, or find that something is holding them back. They often have no trigger to push them into action. They are stuck in the early steps of the change process.

Being afraid of failure will prevent progress. Become aware of what that is for you and learn to release these limiting beliefs.

- Change that fear into a positive opportunity to reach your goal.
- If doubt persists, then try to do the behaviour anyway and see what happens. Even if you get it wrong, you will learn and can try a different way of doing it.
- Overcoming fear leads to personal growth.
- Stop procrastinating.
- Be organised.
- Plan for success.

If you are struggling to get started, then you need to reflect more on your 'why', your values and your dreams, so you can align those with the health goals you need to achieve (see Appendices).

Do your values include being healthy and full of energy? Is this story consistent with you? (See Appendices.)

Then set yourself up for success:

- Start with a one- or two-minute walk
- Do it so you enjoy it
- Have fun trying and then stop
- On the next day, do it again
- Add one minute

- Tell yourself: 'I get to exercise,' instead of 'I have to exercise'. Others may not be able to exercise.
- Be happy, grateful and visualise success already achieved, how that looks and feels and visualise what actions you are already taking to achieve this goal. Do this every day as often as possible.
- A patient of mine told me how he did this by running for five minutes and walking for five minutes once a day for five days and then built that up over weeks. Short intervals of running/walking allow the heart rate to steadily increase and are great for health and energy management.
- Share your stories with other people and learn tips and tricks from each other.
- Track with monitors or apps if you feel this helps.
- Join groups like Nike Run Club or VHI park runs.
- Get an accountability partner. Interact with online running communities or local running clubs.
- Keep focused on achieving your goal. You might have a goal card in your pocket or on your phone that you look at every day.

15

Long-Lasting Health and Happiness

Transforming your heart health happens when you internalise your life's true purpose and you take responsibility for it. To keep your heart in good health requires a balance between vision, purpose, values, physical heart health, behaviour and emotional health, connection, and social community. It requires a healthy, positive mind, focused on taking steps towards being happy and healthy every day. The person with such a mind needs to be:

- Initiative-taking
- Walking regularly
- Eating healthier
- Sleeping better
- Less stressed
- Feeling happy
- Having fun
- Being active with friends, family and community

Finding your purpose, drafting your story and aligning it with your heart health behaviours requires a tailored personal plan. This is possible when you discover:

- Who you really are
- What you want
- Your inner self
- Self-compassion (look after your self-care first)

Being authentic drives healing, growth and gets you practising habits towards permanent health transformation. As you do this, your self-awareness grows, and you can change your thoughts and beliefs to improve your situation. With the right support and coaching you can grow your self-awareness and declare your new health and wellbeing vision to yourself and those around you. This is the ultimate in self-care, and you commit to change and act by changing your unhealthy behaviours and starting new behaviours. You can easily master your vision of being healthier in all aspects of your life. Only you can do the press-ups.

Whole heart health defines your lifespan. Health behaviour change is the route to better health: be it starting or sustaining change or both. People know that poor lifestyle habits adversely impact their health, but they do not know how to change those habits and build new routines. This change is hard. It amounts to time, effort, patience, and persistence, but it can be achieved effortlessly by following the right system. This is how to transform knowing into doing and closing that gap forever.

Poor planning, misunderstanding, lack of support and mind-wandering undo 99 per cent of successful change efforts. This can happen within one week of starting behaviour change. The same happens before change has even started for many people. There will always be difficulties and we all need to accept that and move forward.

Living by your purpose and values, including being the healthiest version of yourself, is the best way to improve your health. You choose what lifestyle behaviours you need to adopt and then take one small step forward each day.

Taking care of your mind and your lifestyle can prevent, treat and reverse many chronic diseases and thereby extend health and life span. How you respond to your perceived life and health circumstances determines how long, healthy and happy your life will be.

Lifestyle medicine is prevention, treatment and potential reversal of chronic disease through a multidisciplinary patient-centred approach. It works. Yet so few people take this medicine. If you want to live a long and healthy life that will only happen by practising healthy life habits every day.

Every longevity study from around the world identifies seven consistent success habits that are needed to have a healthy, happy, long life. Life is to be enjoyed and full of fun for all. Dream big and use your imagination to conjure up your healthy self. See what and how it feels, affirm that with happiness and gratitude and commit by doing to enjoy your personal best health. Get into the habit of:

- Being happy
- Being connected – to family and friends
- Being physically active
- Living with purpose every day
- Healthy eating
- Being calm and taking self-time each day
- Being present in the moment every day

Conclusion

Heart disease is the number one killer and can take someone's life at any age – old or young. Looking after your heart health reduces the risk of premature death.

Lifestyle medicine can prevent, treat and reverse chronic diseases that cause heart disease. The pillars include:

- Not smoking
- Healthy eating
- Physical activity
- Sleep
- Stress management
- Social connection

These pillars account for 80 per cent of chronic diseases and they are all reversible.

The American Heart Association has acknowledged that heart health is determined by these pillars, along with blood pressure, diabetes and cholesterol levels. It identifies that your social determinants (where you live, literacy, education, economics, housing, support, etc.) are contributory. Improving these areas of heart health extends life and reduces all disease risk, even non-heart illnesses like cancer, Alzheimer's disease and lung diseases.

Chronic illness is caused by human behaviour in 50 per cent of cases, social determinants/environment in 20 per cent, genes in

20 per cent and hospital access in 10 per cent. Efforts that focus outside hospital care are likely to have the greatest impact on human health.

Covid-19 has killed millions of people worldwide. Those who have had the worst outcomes have pre-existing chronic medical diseases and/or poor social health circumstances (like over-crowding or poor housing). Sadly, these deaths might have been reduced if being healthy was everyone's priority in life. In those who have survived Covid-19 or who struggle with stress and life, or in those who have had lesser Covid illnesses, the lessons of being healthier are there for everyone to see.

Health is defined by the World Health Organization as social, mental, spiritual, financial, emotional and physical health, and not merely the absence of disease. This requires a broad-minded approach to patient care, such as the Whole Heart Health Model. This addresses purpose, physical and emotional health, and improves health outcomes of patients and caregivers.

Health improvements come from changing human behav-iours such as poor eating habits, inactivity, not sleeping, smoking, drinking too much alcohol and being chronically stressed. Moti-vating change is limited by patients changing their minds. Infor-mation changes nothing. Having real purpose and acting changes everything.

The easiest way to change behaviour is one step at a time. This can be manifested with visualisation, goal-setting, affirma-tions, gratitude and behaviour design. Once the behaviour is easy, enjoyable, fun to do, and aligns with lifestyle issues and your health goal, then prompting a patient to do it should be automatic.

Patients experiment with what works and then they can increase repetitions each day or week. Starting ridiculously small and taking your time is the best approach. Getting into a healthy routine works. Having reminders, appropriate behaviours to improve health and having fun doing the behaviours is essential for the process to work. Behaviour design allows for ways to make the new behaviour easier to do and for it to become habitual.

Long-term health change is aligned with your purpose and aspirations in life. Knowing what you want and why helps you to stick with goals to become healthier even when you may not want to do the behaviours.

Your mind controls your thoughts, feelings and actions. How you respond to those thoughts (positive or negative) will define the actions and subsequent results that you achieve. Being healthy reduces the risk of heart attacks. Sometimes your mind will trick you by bringing up thoughts from your past, like: 'I cannot stop smoking because no programme has ever worked for me.' Reframing those thoughts and training your mind to be less critical and more positive will give you the optimism to achieve success and that will also help you live a longer and happier life.

My approach addresses physical and emotional heart health. It takes a behaviour approach to get to the root of a heart problem. This Whole Heart approach engages patients where they are at and helps them to change heart health by teaching easy, effective and fun ways to become healthier and thereby live long, happy lives. Everyone has the same opportunity to live a long, healthy, happy life.

The future of health needs to change from the current model because it is not working – our health system is overwhelmed and mortality from leading causes like heart disease are not improving. We need to look at the problem in diverse ways or from various positions. The future is about actively listening to patients and getting them involved in their own health care and collaborating with providers and clinicians. One way forward is value-based care that includes patients' values and patients looking after their own health by adopting simple behaviours and sustaining whole heart health habits; by collaborating with community and primary care to stay well and attend for check-ups, screenings and vaccinations; and using hospitals for emergencies only. Giving patients responsibility and rewarding that is also an option. The government in the Czech Republic are paying citizens €50 per month to stop smoking!

Healthier patients will have fewer health care needs, live longer and be more productive. This will enable other people to learn from them and become healthier themselves.

The best medical advice is to be the healthiest version of yourself every day and to take on the identity of being a happy, healthy person by acting in that way too.

APPENDICES

APPENDIX I

SEVEN-MINUTE HEALTH CHECK

- How healthy are you? Do you look after your physical wellbeing?
- Do you smoke? Do you take recreational drugs?
- Do you drink more than twelve small glasses of alcohol per week?
- Do you sleep at least seven to eight hours (uninterrupted) every night?
- Do you take some form of physical activity like a brisk walk for at least 30 minutes per day/150 minutes per week?
- Do you spend time with family and friends?
- Do you eat at least five portions of vegetables every day?
- Do you drink at least six large glasses of water every day?
- Do you visit your doctor for a medical examination every year/ do same through work?
- Do you visit the doctor annually if over the age of 50 years? Have you got a family history of cancer, heart disease or stroke?
- Do you feel stressed/burned out/worthless/depressed at work or home?
- Do you know what you want in life? Have you a mission and purpose?

SUGGESTIONS

Read this list. Take your time. Do this every day for fourteen days.

Write a food diary (record all foods you eat each day for fourteen days and look at what you can change based on your goal, e.g. losing weight).

REFLECT

Where are you now? And where are you trying to get to?

What are you good at already?

APPENDIX 2

WHAT AREA OF YOUR LIFE WOULD YOU LIKE TO WORK ON FIRST?

Please rate where you are in the life areas below by choosing a number from 0 to 10.
  0–4 Dissatisfied
  5 Could be better
  6–7 Reasonable
  8–10 Very satisfied

- Achievements to date
- Work, professional and school life
- Financial freedom
- Home – happy where you live?
- Social status
- Friendships
- Romantic life
- Spirituality
- Family life
- Fun and adventure
- Self-confidence

- Values and principles
- Self-care (me, emotions, physical and psychological)
- Physical health
- Mental health
- Future hopes
- Work-life balance
- Rest and relaxation time
- Making a difference in the world
- General life satisfaction

Take the lowest-scoring area first, and decide on small, concrete steps you can make to improve your happiness/satisfaction in this area. Once you have improved your score in this area, you can move on to the next low-scoring area to address.

APPENDIX 3

Core Values List

- Abundance
- Acceptance
- Achievement
- Adventure
- Affection
- Ambition
- Appreciation
- Approachability
- Balance
- Beauty
- Benevolence
- Bravery
- Brilliance
- Boldness
- Calmness
- Caring
- Charity
- Calmness
- Compassion
- Connection
- Contentment
- Creativity
- Daring
- Discovery
- Diversity
- Eagerness
- Energy
- Excellence
- Family
- Fearlessness
- Fitness
- Frugality
- Fun
- Generosity
- Grace
- Growth
- Happiness
- Health
- Hero
- Humour

- Imagination
- Ingenuity
- Love
- Loyalty
- Making a difference
- Mastery
- Mindfulness
- Meticulousness
- Open-mindedness
- Perfectionism
- Playfulness
- Power
- Pragmatism
- Being present
- Professionalism
- Punctuality
- Recognition
- Relaxation
- Religion
- Resourcefulness
- Rest
- Selflessness
- Service
- Sharing
- Shrewdness
- Silence
- Simplicity
- Sincerity
- Skilfulness
- Soundness
- Spirituality
- Strength
- Sympathetic
- Team
- Thankfulness
- Tidiness
- Trust
- Unity
- Unflappability
- Valour
- Vivaciousness
- Vitality
- Warmth
- Wealth
- Wisdom
- Wonder
- Youthfulness
- Zest

Use these values to define what is important to you. Pick two or three.

What gives you energy? Pick an energy level of 0–10.

Reflect on how your values align with your vision and goals in life and health.

Do they match or not?

Consider re-engineering your goals and vision to your values if there is a mismatch.

(Check online for other values that may not be listed here.)

APPENDIX 4

Whole Heart Health Model

Me: Vision, aspirations, purpose, intentions and goals

MY LIFESTYLE PILLARS AND MY SELF-CARE

- Physical activity
- Environment – physical and emotional
- Power of mind – healing and relaxing; fun and happiness
- Spirit and soul – growth and connection
- Family, friends, co-workers – relationships
- Recharge – sleep, refresh
- Food – nourish and fuel
- Personal development – personal and work life
- Stress reduction
- Professional care – medical/physical health
- My community – people and groups

WHAT ARE YOUR ASPIRATIONS? YOUR VISION? WHAT MATTERS TO YOU? FOR WHAT DO YOU LIVE?

- Physical activity – movement, exercise, walking, lifting, bending, balance
- Surroundings – home, outside, work, clutter, nature
- Power of mind – thoughts, beliefs, mindset. Mindfulness, tapping, relaxation response, tai chi, meditation
- Spirit and soul – connect with something greater than yourself, purpose, nature, art, music, spirit.
- Family/friends/co-workers/a pet – positive, friendly, supportive, fun.
- Recharge – sleep for eight hours, enjoy your day and refresh, take a break.
- Food/healthy eating – small portions; more vegetables, fish, plants, water; less alcohol
- Personal development – what brings joy to your home and work life?
- Stress reduction – optimism and positivity, growth mindset, open and creative, energetic
- Professional care – prevention, taking an active role in your own health

REFLECT

What is your vision of your best self? What would your life look like? What would you be doing? Immerse yourself and practice visualisation using the time travel technique (imagining your future and travelling back to now, visualising what you need to do to achieve this). Are there any areas that you would like to work on and where might you start? Reach out to a friend/doctor and talk about this with them.

Selected References

Benson, Herbert (1975) *The Relaxation Response*, New York, NY: Harper Collins.

Boles, D., De Sousa, M., Turnwald, B.P., Hori, R., Duarte, T., Zahrt O.H., Markus, H.R. and Crum, A.J. (2021) 'Can Exercise and Eating Healthy Be Fun and Indulgent instead of Boring and Depriving? Targeting Mindsets about the Process of Engaging in Healthy Behaviours', *Frontiers in Psychology*, October, Volume 12.

Fleet, Thurman (2000) *Rays of Dawn: Natural Laws of the Body, Mind and Soul*, San Antonio, TX: Concept-Therapy Institute.

Fogg, B.J. (2020) *Tiny Habits: Why Starting Small Makes Lasting Change Easy*, London: Virgin Books

Frates, Beth; Bonnet, Jonathan P.; Joseph, Richard; Peterson, James A. (2019) *The Lifestyle Medicine Handbook: An Introduction to the Power of Healthy Habits*, Monterey, CA: Healthy Learning.

Global Cardiovascular Risk Consortium et al. (2023) 'Global Effect of Modifiable Risk Factors on Cardiovascular Disease and Mortality', *New England Journal of Medicine*, October, 5(389): 1273–1285.

Goddard, Neville (2022) *The Power of Awareness* and *Feeling Is the Secret* (double edition), Wescombe Publishing.

Haanel, Charles (2020) *The Master Key System*, New York: G&D Media.

Hill, Napoleon (Edited by Arthur Pell) (2004) *Think and Grow Rich*, London: Vermillion.

Irish Heart Foundation, www.irishheart.ie.

Kenny, R.A. et al. (2010–2023) *The Irish Longtitudinal Study on Ageing* (TILDA), various publications, www.tilda.ie.

Lloyd Jones, D., Allen, N., Anderson, C., Black, T., Brewer, L., Foraker, R., Grandner, M., Lavretsky, H., Perak, A.M., Sharma, G., Rosamond, W. and on behalf of the American Heart Association (2022) 'Life's Essential 8: Updating and Enhancing the American Heart Association's Construct of Cardiovascular Health: A Presidential Advisory From the American Heart Association', *Circulation*, 146(5): e18–e43.

Maltz, Maxwell (2023) *PsychoCybernetics*, London: Souvenir Press.

Mensah, G., Fuster, V. and Roth, G.A. (2023) 'A Heart-Healthy and Stroke-Free World: Using Data to Inform Global Action', *Journal of the American College of Cardiology*, 8(25): 2343–2349.

Murphy, Joseph (2011) *The Power of the Subconscious Mind*, London: Penguin Publishing Group.

Omstead, Janet (2019) *The Play Book: How to Get in the Habit of Good Health*, Janetomstead.com.

Prochaska, James and Prochaska, Janice M. (2016) *Changing to Thrive: Using the Stages of Change to Overcome the Top Threats to Your Health and Happiness*, Center City, MN: Hazelden Publishing.

Swart, Tara (2020) *The Source: Open Your Mind, Change Your Life*, London: Vermilion.

US Department of Veterans Affairs, *Whole Health Model of Care*, www.va.gov/wholehealth.

Health Improvement and Heart Attack Prevention Programmes

Dr Robert Kelly, MD MBA FRCPI FESC FACC, Cardiology and Lifestyle Medicine Coaching

Supported by novel AI-based continued learning and education tools. Available worldwide with details below.

I run online self-paced video-based learning programmes to help you improve health and prevent heart attacks happening for the first and second time.

The programmes run over eight weeks of weekly Zoom-based group calls where I coach the group and help you to apply the video-based learning to improve your heart health, prevent heart attacks and live longer.

The content addresses mindset, goal setting, health behaviours and building new health habits to achieve your goals, such as avoiding a heart attack. I apply the pillars of lifestyle medicine that are explained in this book to your life and help you to make changes one pillar and one step at a time.

The biggest challenge for everyone is that most of us know what to do but few people do anything about their personal health, even after having had a cardiac event.

My programmes will help you to remove those barriers between knowing and doing. They will give you all the necessary tools and coach you exactly in how to turn around and permanently transform your heart health. Many of these principles are discussed in this book.

www.drrobertkelly.ie